2 BIG

MEASUREMENT, CAUSES, HAZARDS AND TREATMENT OF OBESITY

Randall Travis, MD

ACKNOWLEDGEMENTS

My thanks to the following persons who have reviewed all or part of the manuscript: Laura Travis, Greg Norris, Sandra Chetnik, Robert Johnson,and Arthur Kern.

I owe a special debt of gratitude to Julie Kitchell who prepared the manuscript for publication.

Randall H. Travis MD

2 BIG: MEASUREMENT, CAUSES, HAZARDS AND TREATMENT OF OBESITY
by Randall Travis, MD

ISBN-10: 0981685013

ISBN-13: 978-0981685014

Published March 2011 by ImageRe: Digital Works   http://www.imagere.com

Printed by: createspace   http://createspace.com

TABLE OF CONTENTS

PROLOGUE

In 1997 Medlars, the computerized data base of the National Library of Medicine, listed 860 reviews of the subject "obesity" in the biomedical publications in English alone since 1966. By 2008 the number had increased to 4670. It seems that nearly every issue of the printed mass media includes an article on the subject. Advertisements abound offering corrective action, for a price.

In this setting why would anyone want to add to the flood of printed paper concerning this problem? The reason is that much of what has been published is false, misleading, or uninformed. This has been true not only of material intended for the general public but also of material intended for the several kinds of practicing professionals who serve people concerned about body fat. It has consisted largely of largely futile exhortations to diet and exercise, with variations of added psychotherapy and drugs, but providing few of the established facts increasingly available.

On the other hand, the writings of scholars and research scientists have reflected a quite different perspective, rational and consistent with established facts. It seemed to me that there was a need for a text intended both for the general public and for the physicians, dietitians, and exercise specialists who work with people concerned about body fat. This monograph was written thinking of the educated general reader and of the professional who wants a critical overview of the science related to the subject but without a heavy burden of detail and mathematics. The sections entitled **APPENDIX 1** and **APPENDIX 2** contain explanations and supplemental material for those with an appetite for more information. Topics are arranged alphabetically.

For the benefit of the professionals there is a select citation of sources. I have attempted, where appropriate, to confine citations to peer-reviewed publications. Internet references have been usually avoided as a consequence of their tendency to disappear [1]. No attempt has been made to provide a comprehensive reference list for any topic but rather to give one or two citations which would provide a trail to the remainder of the relevant literature for interested persons. If I have failed to choose, from among many, a reference which for some reason should have priority, I apologize. The literature of this field provides an embarrassment of riches.

Nearly all of the references cited are available free in some form to anyone with an internet connection at *http://www.ncbi.nlm.nih.gov/entrez/query.fcgi*.

The United States, almost alone among advanced industrialized nations, has failed to adopt the metric system of weights and measures and has clung to the archaic pound-foot system. This is a serious failing as demonstrated by the 1999 Mars spacecraft fiasco in which pound-foot data were confused with metric data in programming the Climate Orbiter with the result that the craft was lost. Consequently whenever I have cited pound-foot data I have included the metric equivalents in parentheses.

CHAPTER ONE: INTRODUCTION

Despite public interest and, increasingly, alarm in both public and private sectors for more than a half-century there has been a relentless increase in overweight and obesity revealed by the following sampling of publications readily available in the U.S.:

- *1953 publication*

    "The increase in mortality accompanying obesity justifies, it seems, calling obesity the "Number One Nutrition Problem" and perhaps even the "Number One Public Health Problem" in Western Countries at the present time" [2].

- *1965 publication*

    "That obesity is on the increase, particularly in men and in children and adolescents, is suggested by data from the Selective Service, from the U. S. Public Health Service, and from our own work in suburban school children in the Boston area. For example, the latter suggest a 20 percent increase in prevalence of obesity in the school system of Newton (Mass.) in the last decade" [3].

- *1994 publication*

    "In the period 1988 to 1991, 33.4% of US adults were estimated to be overweight. Comparisons of the 1988 to 1991 overweight prevalence estimates with data from earlier surveys indicate dramatic increases in all race/sex groups. Overweight prevalence increased 8% between the 1976 to 1980 and 1988 to 1991 surveys" [4].

- *2000 publication*

    "The prevalence of obesity increased in the United States through the 1980s. The authors examined 10-year aging and secular (time-related) trends in the Coronary Artery Risk Development in Young Adults (CARDIA) study for indications of whether these trends are continuing…CARDIA is a population-based, prospective study of 5,115 African-American and White men and women aged 18-30 years at baseline. Body weight and overweight prevalence were measured at five time points from 1985-1986 to 1995-96. Statistical treatment allowed partitioning weight gain into that due to secular trends and that due to aging Prevalence of overweight increased markedly and prevalence of severe obesity doubled in all race-sex groups" [5].

- *2006 publication*

    "The prevalence of overweight among children and adolescents and obesity among men increased significantly during the 6-year period from 1999 to 2004; among women, no overall increases in the prevalence of obesity were observed" [6].

- *2008 publication*

    "More than two-thirds of adults and one-third of children in America are obese or at risk for obesity. To reverse this epidemic, we must identify the policy and environmental changes that lead to increased physical activity and better nutrition. We also must support the advocacy that will result in widespread adoption of those policies." Report of the Robert Wood Johnson Foundation available at www.rwjf.org

More recently the phenomena of epidemic overweight and obesity and concern about them have occurred globally as documented by the following quotations from the medical literature:

- *1995 publication*

"Department of Health Statistics show that the prevalence of serious obesity doubled in Britain between 1980 and 1991 and is continuing to increase" [7].

- *1999 publication*

"In the German National Health Interview and Examination Survey 1998 several anthropometric data were obtained from 7124 men and women, aged 18-79 years. These data were analyzed and compared with 1990/92 survey data....the prevalence of overweight ranges from 52% for West German women to 67% for West German men, and of obesity from 18% for West German men to 24.5% for East German women....In the male population, aged 25-69 years, the prevalence of obesity increased by 5.9% in the East and by 11.5% in the West during the past decade. Among females the prevalence of obesity increased by 6.4% in the West but decreased by 6.3% in the East. Still obesity is more prevalent among East German females" [8].

- *1999 publication*

"The term 'epidemic' of obesity implies that obesity is a characteristic of populations, not only of individuals. ...Trends in overweight or obesity among adults showed considerable variability internationally. Some countries including Canada, Finland (men), New Zealand, the United Kingdom, the United States, and Western Samoa showed large increases in prevalence (> 5 percentage points) whereas several other countries showed smaller or no increases" [9].

- *2006 publication*

"WHO's latest projections indicate that globally in 2005: Approximately 1.6 billion adults (age 15+) were overweight; and at least 400 million adults were obese. WHO further projects that by 2015, approximately 2.3 billion adults will be overweight and more than 700 million will be obese.

At least 20 million children under the age of 5 years are overweight globally in 2005.

Once considered a problem only in high-income countries, overweight and obesity are now dramatically on the rise in low- and middle-income countries, particularly in urban settings" [10].

Above are expressions of alarm by researchers from 1953 onward. Probably even earlier statements of concern could be found. For at least fifty five years there has been a relentless increase in the prevalence of obesity in the industrialized world, especially the United States. There is some good news. Data from a November 2007 publication indicate that in recent years there has been a plateau in the increasing prevalence of obesity in US adults. A study examining the trend in prevalence of obesity in American adults 1999-2008 found a reduction in the rate of increasing prevalence with no change in prevalence during the last three years of the study [11]. This finding can be interpreted as indicating some success in public and/or private efforts to control obesity and/or a demonstration that those persons susceptible to obesity are already obese [12].

Ironically there is more good news from Asia and the western hemisphere. Previously the problem attracting most attention was under-nutrition. As prosperity has brought about trends toward western diet and sedentary life there has been a change of emphasis from under-nutrition to over-nutrition. Formerly overweight and obesity were most prevalent in the higher socioeconomic strata. Recently there has been a trend to greater prevalence of overweight and obesity in the lower socioeconomic strata [13;14].

In addition to the psychosocial pain, the costs in human misery in consequence of increased susceptibility to disease and death from **Diabetes Mellitus**, (see **APPENDIX 2**) cardiovascular disease and a long list of other horrors is almost beyond imagining. A whole chapter of this document is devoted to the health consequences of obesity. The economic costs have been estimated in tens of billions of dollars in the United States. "Increases in the proportion of ... spending on obese people relative to people of normal weight account for 27 percent of the rise in inflation-adjusted per capita spending between 1987 and 2001..."[15]. While this has been occurring there has developed in the United States a huge industry offering "treatment" of obesity, which has been, from the epidemiological perspective, almost totally ineffective. This document is written for the purpose of enlarging public understanding of the problem, resulting in continuing support of research, our best hope for solution, and, in any case, a common sense, fact-guided coping. Not least among benefits, would be a more humane, more understanding, more compassionate public attitude toward obese persons.

We must not fail to be aware that although the problems presented by the prevalence of obesity in the industrialized world are not trivial they are dwarfed by the global prevalence of under-nutrition. Worldwide there are more than 800 million undernourished people, nearly all in developing and transitional countries, including more than 180 million children under the age of 10 years. The children are at risk of maldevelopment and of becoming impaired adults [16;17].

CHAPTER TWO: HOW IS OBESITY MEASURED?

To describe someone as obese, in common speech, is to make an esthetic and, sometimes, moral judgment based on body conformation. As in other esthetic judgments there is great variation in opinion: from time-to-time, by the same person; within groups, ethnic, national, gender, or age-related; and in historical periods of time. It is always pejorative. Synonyms are, "big", "corpulent", "overweight", "fleshy", "heavy", "stout", and "fat". The latter expression is closest to the medical and scientific definition.

In medical and scientific writing, to describe someone as obese is understood to mean that the person has an excessive amount of body fat. This definition immediately suggests two questions:
How much body fat is an excessive amount?
How is the amount of body fat measured?

The biomedical professionals concerned about this question assume that an amount of body fat is excessive when it enhances risk to health. On the other hand, most people in the general population concerned about their body fat are concerned about their appearance. This subject will be discussed in the chapter entitled "Medical Hazards of Obesity". It has begun to seem likely that our interest in total body fat as an indicator and mediator of health risk has been overemphasized. It seems possible that equally or more important is the amount and metabolic activity of regional fat deposits, especially intra-abdominal fat.

Measurements of body constituents, including fat, do not have the precision, specificity, and reproducibility found in the exact physical sciences, physics and chemistry. In fact, it is generous to call some of the reported values estimates. Nevertheless, both practice and theory depend upon quantitative data in this field as in every science-related field.

In the research much attention has been focused on two quantities, "fat component", and "fat-free component". Early in the systematic study of body composition following World War II, "fat component" came to be the designation of that quantity of fat which could be extracted by a suitable solvent during direct chemical analysis of the whole body of a human or animal ("chemical fat"). "Fat-free component" was the residuum after extraction of the fat. Arithmetically fat- free component was the difference between total body weight and the fat component. At that time the expression "lean body mass" referred to an estimate of fat-free component accomplished by some indirect means in the intact human, e.g. by densitometry, to be discussed below [18] and in **APPENDIX 1**. Subsequently some authors have used the expressions "lean body mass" and "fat-free component" as synonyms. Some authors recently use the expression "lean body mass" to refer to the entity of fat-free component less bone mineral content. The terminology of study of human body composition tends to be confusing and these distinctions are more important to the research community than the general readership.

Clearly, "fat component" is not synonymous with "adipose tissue", as some authors have assumed. A typical example of adipose tissue is the fatty tissue underlying the skin of everyone. Another example is the fatty deposits found among the viscera of the abdomen. It is correct that most of the fat component in most people is contained in the adipose tissue though there is some fat in muscle and liver. However, adipose tissue is a cellular material containing, in addition to fat, a fat-free element consisting of the supporting structures of cells and the cell contents, including water, proteins, carbohydrates, nucleic acids, and minerals, all of which are part of the fat-free component. Adipose tissue also includes an extracellular space containing water, proteins, and minerals. In addition to fat-containing cells, adipocytes, adipose tissue contains blood vessels and numerous macrophages, cells of the immune system.

Direct chemical analyses of whole bodies have been made most frequently in animals, fetuses, and infants, but also in a small number of adults. The first reports concerning such studies were published by German investigators as early as 1859. The number of adult human bodies so examined has been too few to provide insight into the processes which determine human body composition. However, the values for various constituents thus obtained have been important in the design and development of indirect means of estimation of components of body composition. Although direct chemical analysis of whole bodies is the most reliable means of obtaining accurate information about body composition, there has been little activity in this line of investigation recently. The practical obstacles are overwhelming. Permission must be obtained from families, and sometimes officers of the law. Suitable bodies, free of confounding disease, and not too badly damaged by the processes of dying are seldom available. Special apparatus is needed. Finally, there is what the eminent researcher Elsie Widdowson called "the most serious trouble of all--one's distaste for the whole business" [19]. Other authors may or may not have intended black humor with the remark that "post-mortem desiccation of cadavers ...has no practical significance in clinical investigation" [20].

An ideal measurement of human body composition would be specific, accurate, highly reproducible, inexpensive, readily portable, and would require little training or practice for satisfactory use. It would allow for a valid determination of body composition independent of age, gender, ethnicity/race, and disease, or unusual characteristics, e.g. extreme obesity. This ideal has not been found.

Uses for suitable methods of assessing human body composition, and specifically fat-free component and fat component, include studies in epidemiology, nutrition, metabolism, physiology, and even assessment of benefits of individuals in weight loss programs. Would you like to know whether your five pound weight loss was all fat, no fat, or partly fat?

Many methods have been developed for estimating body fat, many of them ingenious, elegant. They are briefly reviewed below and reviewed in detail in **APPENDIX 1**.

They can be divided into methods predominantly used for research and physiological investigations and those predominantly used for clinical and epidemiological purposes. Perhaps unfortunately the research methods have been largely abandoned by clinical investigators who presently rely almost entirely on the Body Mass Index, a deeply flawed clinical method.

RESEARCH METHODS

Densitometry ("Underwater Weighing")

"Under water weighing", sometimes called densitometry, is accomplished by first weighing the subject in air and then completely immersed in water. The subsequent calculation of fat component and fat-free component depends upon assumptions about the specific density of those two components and is therefore subject to errors. The procedure is uncomfortable, frightening to many people, and not suitable for children. It was among the first methods used and has been employed as a criterion method, the "gold standard" (for details see **APPENDIX 1**).

Dual Energy X-Ray Absorptiometry ("DEXA")

Dual energy X-ray absorptiometry has been used to estimate body composition, based on the differential absorption of two beams of x-rays of different energy by fat, bone, and other tissues. The machines required are widely available for estimation of bone density, especially in people who have or are at risk for osteoporosis. In that role they have been very popular.

Studies in pigs in which estimates of fat by dual x-ray absorptiometry were compared with fat determined by direct chemical analysis of carcasses have raised questions about the validity of the dual x-ray estimates [21-29] (for details, see **APPENDIX 1**).

Four Component Model

The four component model is an example of what can be called generically the multicomponent model. In this model independent measurements of separate components are made by combinations of the above methods and the results are mathematically integrated to yield a value for total body fat or some other desired value. For example, one Four-component model is based on measurement of body density as described above, total body water by isotope dilution, and total body bone ash by dual energy X-ray absorptiometry [30-32]. The calculation of body fat by this means is outlined in **APPENDIX 1**. Many assumptions are required for the calculations, some of them not well established.

Impedance

Impedance, sometimes called bioelectrical impedance, as an index of the fat and fat-free components is estimated by attaching electrodes to wrists and ankles and passing an imperceptible electric current through the body, measuring the impedance, a property of electrical resistance. In the calculation of fat and fat-free components it is assumed that impedance is an index of body water, present in constant proportion in the fat-free component. Knowing the amount of body water and the fraction of fat-free component which is water allows calculation of the fat-free component. The fat component is the difference between the body weight and the fat-free component.

Unfortunately, human bodies have complex electrical properties and water is not a constant fraction of the fat-free component. Estimates of body composition have not been satisfactorily concordant with estimates by densitometry (see **APPENDIX 1**).

Neutron Activation Analysis

When certain naturally occurring elements in the human body are subjected to bombardment with neutrons they emit a characteristic secondary radiation which can be measured and can be the basis for an estimate of the amount of the element in the body. This principle has been applied to measurement of carbon, nitrogen, calcium, phosphorous and chlorine in living humans. Total body fat can be estimated by first measuring total body carbon and nitrogen. If the proportion of fat which is carbon is assumed and the proportion of protein which is carbon and the proportion of protein which is nitrogen are assumed, it is possible to calculate an estimate of total fat. Some measurements have been made but utilization and even evaluation have been limited by concerns about the exposure of subjects to radiation. Further it is recognized that assumptions about the proportions of carbon and nitrogen in various tissues are at best approximations (see **APPENDIX 1**).

Total Potassium

Total body potassium was measured by principles of isotope dilution using the naturally occurring radioactive isotope of potassium, ^{40}K. Assuming a constant concentration of potassium in the fat-free component, the size of the fat-free component was easily calculated. However, measurement of the small amount of potassium which is ^{40}K is very difficult; requiring complex expensive machines and this technique also has never been used much (see **APPENDIX 1**).

Total Exchangable Potassium

Total exchangeable potassium has been used as a measure of body composition by employment of the principles of isotope dilution (see **APPENDIX 1**). The Atomic Energy Commission made available to biomedical investigators a radioactive form of potassium, ^{42}K, not found in nature. If certain assumptions about body potassium were correct, ^{42}K could be used to estimate the size of the fat-free component. It was soon discovered that the radioactive potassium was contaminated with radioactive substances which were not potassium and the assumptions concerning the behavior of potassium in the body were incorrect. Consequently this procedure never gained much popularity.

Summary

The above-described research-type methods for indirect estimates of components of body composition all have two features in common. Firstly, none has been rigorously validated, i.e. shown to measure with acceptable, or at least known accuracy what they are purported to measure, especially fat. The ultimate validating procedure is chemical analysis of whole bodies. This is unlikely ever to be done. Secondly, all the methods discussed require in their calculations of body fat one or more assumptions which are, at best, approximations of average values in some population. For example, most authors in calculating the weight of the fat-free component, and the fat component, have assumed that the fat-free component is 73% water. In studies in which, in the same individual, total body water was measured by isotope dilution and the mass of the fat-free component was measured either by densitometry or other techniques the fraction of fat-free mass calculated to be water ranged from 68.2% to 78.4%[31;33]. This variation represents both measurement error and biologic variability. The presence of variation of this magnitude necessitates a conclusion that a single measurement in one individual has a large possibility of error, making the value of limited use. However, measurements in large populations may be useful. It is by means of population studies that the methods described above have generated some consensus as a consequence of the amount and consistency of data concerning certain findings, despite the uncertainties.

It is generally accepted that in representative populations:

•people with large fat deposits tend not only to have increased fat but also an increased fat-free component [34];

•weight loss, mediated by dietary caloric restriction, tends to result in loss not only of fat but also of fat-free mass [35;36];

•growth hormone replacement in populations of adults with adult-onset growth hormone deficiency results in an average loss of total body fat, loss of intra-abdominal fat, increased muscle volume, and increased total body water [37-40];

•similar results have been found in populations of obese people not growth hormone deficient [34;41-44] but only with large doses [45];

•the average gain in body weight occurring in both men and women during aging is almost entirely attributable to increased body fat and increased percentage of body weight which is fat [46];

•at all ages, populations of females have an average higher percentage body fat than comparable populations of males [47].

In this abundance of studies in which fat, specifically, has been estimated there seems to have been only limited attempts to define excessive fat. This should not be surprising. Excessive by what standard? By the standard of current fashion? By the standard of health risk? The former standard is the preoccupation of most dieters; the latter is the preoccupation of most professionals concerned about body fat.

All of the above methods of estimating the amount of body fat require expenditure of much time by skilled personnel and the availability of large expensive machines. There is need for methods which can be used in the clinic, in the physicians' office, in the varied sites in which population surveys are performed, and perhaps, some day, in an orbiting space station.

CLINICAL METHODS

Body Mass Index

The use of indices, ratios of weight/height, has a long history in the effort to evaluate body composition, "body build", adiposity. The reasons for the appeal of such an index are obvious. The necessary measurements are easily made, are frequently routinely made, and can be acceptably accurate. Several indices have been used at various times: weight/height (W/H), weight/height squared (W/H^2), cube root of weight/height ($W^{1/3}/H$), weight/height cubed (W/H^3), and height/cube root of weight ($H/W^{1/3}$). The index most widely used at this time is W/H^2, known for a century as Quetelet's index in recognition of the French investigator who first calculated it. In 1972 Keys [48] suggested that it be called the body mass index (BMI) and so it is today.

The BMI has come to have an important presence in the writing about the clinical aspects of body fat. Numerous epidemiological studies have reported it as the principal datum of evaluation of body composition. In 1998 the National Heart, Lung, and Blood Institute, in a clinical guideline, recommended the BMI as the principal basis for a conclusion of excess adiposity in individuals. This perhaps may be the best possible public policy but it is not necessarily good science and it is not necessarily good clinical practice.

Serious investigations of the properties of the various indices of weight began in 1962 [49]. A desirable index would have: 1) little correlation with height, and 2) high correlation with weight. These requirements assume that, in a population, the distribution of adiposity will be the same in tall people as short people. Satisfaction of these requirements would allow useful comparisons of tall persons with short persons. For persons of the same height but different weights, the index value should reflect the differing weights.

By those criteria survey results of populations of both men and women in the United States, Europe, Africa and Asia indicate that, for men, the body mass index (BMI, W/H^2) is generally the best of the indices considered, with usually little correlation with height and substantial correlation with weight. However, not all surveys have indicated a satisfyingly low correlation with height and this is seldom evaluated in reports describing the body mass index of populations. Correlations with weight range from good to modest in various reports. For women, many reports indicate that the ratio weight/height (W/H) better satisfies the requirements of little correlation with height and good correlation with weight. However, in the interest of comparability between different studies the conventional index, W/H^2, is usually the datum reported for women.

Defining overweight and obesity in children has been difficult. Ideal standards would be based on adiposity-related morbidities and/or adiposity-related morbidities developing later in adulthood. Adiposity-related morbidities are not common in children although some significant prevalences have appeared in adolescents and data concerning childhood obesity as a risk factor for adult morbidity are limited [12;50]. Difficulty is enhanced by the facts that medians for BMI, the most commonly used index of adiposity, vary with age and gender and vary differently in different national populations [51]. Consequently establishing age- and gender-specific cutoff points for overweight and obesity has a definitely arbitrary nature.

The United States government Center for Disease Control and Prevention has promulgated growth charts for children in which body mass index for age and gender are presented as percentiles 5th, 85th, and 95th, for ages two to 20 years. The data used to construct the charts have been obtained from periodic surveys of American children. Clinicians have been advised to use these charts for evaluation of obesity in children. Those exceeding the 85th percentile are said to be overweight, and those exceeding the 95th percentile are said to be obese. The charts are available at: *http://www.cdc.gov/nchs/about/major/nhanes/growthcharts/clinical_charts.htm* (accessed 06/08/09). The charts have been revised as new data has become available. There is a risk that we will see an Orwellian progression in which, as American children become fatter, they seem no worse and children in starving areas of the world seem steadily worse.

The World Health Organization has developed international standards for child overweight and obesity based on measurements in six countries, given optimal nutrition and health. There is concern that the standards may not be entirely appropriate for American children. Details are available at *http://www.who.int/childgrowth/mgrs/en/* (accessed 06/08/09). The standards were developed for the purpose of making comparisons between nations and cultures over time. For that purpose they have provided interesting and plausible information.

There are serious concerns about the mathematical properties of the W/H^2 ratio and about what conclusions regarding body composition are permissible based exclusively on that ratio [52;53] (see **Body Mass Index** in **APPENDIX 1**.) The mathematical properties of the index are such that it is suspected that the prevalence of obesity, in adults, tends to be underestimated in tall people and overestimated in short people [54].

There has been since the earliest recorded descriptions of weight for height ratios a persistent tendency to present them as "indices of adiposity". Clearly, they cannot be exactly that but are indices of body weight. However, body weight is not unrelated to body fat which is one of many components of body weight including bone, water, and muscle. The nature of the body mass index means that it cannot have a simple one-to-one relationship to fat mass. Attempts to evaluate a simple correlation between body mass index and total body fat or percent body fat , estimated by densitometry, total body potassium, or total body water in adults, have ranged from barely significant to excellent [48;55-62]. Perhaps the range of results reflects not only the variety of criterion measurements but also the diversity of populations studied with respect to gender, age, and race. There is now a suspicion that use of the body mass index without consideration for gender, age, and "ethnicity/ race" is inappropriate in children. Comparisons within relatively homogeneous groups may be useful but comparisons between groups and comparisons of children of different ages are unreliable and estimates of fat content of individual children are probably subject to large errors [63].

The recommendation of the National Institutes of Health that the body mass index be taken as the basis for a diagnosis of obesity in an individual adult should be received with caution. The expert panel which formulated the recommendations defined overweight as a body mass index of 25 to 29.9 and an index of 30 or greater as obesity. At a typical height of 6 ft (183 cm) a man with a body mass index of 25 weighs 184 lb (83 kg). An index of 27 for that person indicates a weight of 199 lb (90 kg) and an index 30 is associated with a weight of 227 lb (100 kg). For a typical woman of stature 5 ft 2 in, 62 in (157 cm), an index of 25 computes to a body weight of 136 lb (62 kg), an index of 27 to a weight of 147 lb (67 kg), and an index of 30 to a body weight of 164 lb (74 kg). Allowing an intermediate range of 25 to 29.9 in the index is consistent with a view that the body mass index should be considered a screen for the diagnosis of obesity. If there is any doubt, additional data should be obtained. Examples of useful additional data are abdominal girth, family history, personal weight history, presence of metabolic or cardiovascular risk factors, life style, and the regional body distribution of visible fat.

To illustrate the hazards of excessive reliance on the body mass index contrast two men. Both are 5 ft 8 in (1.74 m) tall and both weigh 166.5 lb (75 kg) and consequently both have a body mass index of 25. Rugged Roger, 20 years old, has a thick neck, sloping shoulders, a washboard abdomen and bulging biceps. He is a college wrestler. Ragged Roger, his father, is 70 years old, has a protuberant abdomen, a double chin, and thin arms and legs. He is a retired clerical worker. By densitometry, Rugged Roger has a total body fat content of 6.7 lb (3 kg) and Ragged Roger has a total body fat content of 51.8 lb (23.3 kg).It can appropriately be argued that this example is both extreme and obvious. These are not fictitious data. They are values reported in the literature [55;64]. However, it is an illustration of the fact that the index is most dependable in comparing individuals within a population in which individuals vary little in any characteristic except their body fat content.
Despite its faults, the index has been seen as an indispensable tool in epidemiology for the reason that it not only may provide the only available data relevant to body fat content but the only relevant data which *can* be obtained. Caution is mandatory and mistakes are not only possible but probably are more frequent than we know. Wang and collaborators [65] recruited, by advertising, self-described populations of "whites" and of "Asians" of similar age and gender distributions. For both genders, the "whites" had a higher average body mass index and, by dual photon absorptiometry, lower average percentage body fat. The findings illustrate the difficulties encountered with uncritical use of the ratios, body mass index and percentage body fat.

A very serious effort to supplement or supplant the BMI has been made by analyzing a large data base in which Americans were classified by gender, age 8 to 85, and ethnicity, white, black, and Mexican-American. Fat mass was estimated by dual X-ray absorptiometry and Fat Mass/Height^2 computed. It remains to be seen whether the extra effort and expense of dual X-ray absorptiometry is justified by results in medical and epidemiological work [66]. Perhaps this index is a more accurate index of excess adiposity than the BMI.

Skin Folds

Although measurement of the thickness of skin folds was of sufficient interest to inspire a French investigator to describe a special caliper for the purpose as early as 1890 [35] and there was much study in many lands it was not until 1974 that Durnin and Womersley at the University of Glasgow described a procedure which was widely adopted [67]. A fold of skin is lifted between thumb and forefinger, a caliper applied, and the thickness of the skin fold recorded. In the studies of Durnin and

Womersley four skin folds (biceps, triceps, subscapular, and suprailiac) were measured in 209 men and 272 women ranging in age from 16 years to 72 years and in weight from 94 lb (42.3 kg) to 270 lb (121.5 kg). The final outcome of their labor was a table in which, knowing the sum of measurements of four skin folds, the gender, and the age of the subject, one could find the body fat content as a percentage of body weight. Briefly, the sum of skin folds was used to "predict" whole body density from which percentage body fat was calculated by the Siri equation discussed in the presentation of Densitometry in **APPENDIX 1**. Some aspects of the mathematics and procedures by which measurements of the thickness of Skin folds are used to predict densitometric percent body fat are discussed in the **APPENDIX 1**.

Obviously measurement of skin folds to estimate body fat by estimation of body density has the difficulties associated with densitometry, discussed above, plus the difficulties peculiar to the skin fold technology. Some investigators have found difficulty obtaining consistent measurements. Others have proclaimed that intraobserver variation and interobserver variation can be confined within acceptable limits by careful training and practice. However, even if acceptable measurements can be obtained there are serious grounds for skepticism. The thickness of the skin fold presumably reflects the thickness of the skin plus the thickness of the subcutaneous fat. There is an assumption that the thickness of the subcutaneous fat has a predictable relationship to whole body density and therefore to total body fat. It is clear from the work of many investigators that the relationship is modulated by age, gender, and degree of adiposity [58]. Despite the limitations, measurement of thickness of skin folds continues to be used in various forms because it can be used in clinical settings and at sites of surveys where large and expensive apparatus is inappropriate or impossible. A powerful asset of this technique is that it is one of the very few which can be used in children.

Tables

Evaluation of body weight and, inferentially, adiposity has been frequently based on tables of weight for height, with separate tables by gender and sometimes gender and age. Such tables have been available from the Metropolitan Life Insurance Company since 1912. The values have been characterized as "standard", "desirable", "ideal", "suggested", "recommended" or "acceptable". Sources of such tables in the recent past have been the United States Department of Agriculture in addition to the Metropolitan Life Insurance Company. The most influential have been those published by the Metropolitan Life Insurance Company, most recently in 1983. Although these tables have been used widely they have been severely criticized on two grounds. Firstly, the weights described are "desirable" because they are associated with the lowest mortality in people who buy life insurance. There is under-representation of the poor, minorities, and women. Secondly, separate ranges were recommended for persons of small, medium, or large frame. No definition of frame size was given and no method of ascertaining the frame size of an individual was described. Some efforts were made to define frame size by measurements of shoulder width, chest width, ankle or knee width etc. but no consensus was ever achieved. Consequently, classification of the weight of an individual on the basis of the tables can be to some extent whatever anyone chooses for whatever reason to make it.

CHAPTER THREE: CAUSES OF OBESITY

ADVANCE ADVICE

Although this chapter is entitled "CAUSES OF OBESITY", it does not conclusively describe the causes of obesity. They are largely unknown. The chapter does describe modern research findings which may eventually lead to knowledge of the causes of obesity and solutions for the problems associated with obesity. If you are not interested in the activities of scientists working in this field you may want to skip this chapter and go on to chapters four and five, entitled "MEDICAL HAZARDS OF OBESITY" and "TREATMENT".

However, if you are one of the numerous people who have tried multiple remedies, diets, exercise, psychotherapy, drugs, alternative medicine, and prayer, without sustained success, you may find both comfort and hope in the assurances in this chapter that obesity is not a moral lapse. Comfort because you have been stigmatized, stereotyped, shunned and exploited although your worst offense is being born with a constellation of genes which are unfavorable in an environment of abundant food and minimum incentive to physical exertion. Hope because modern research may provide a better future for obese people than they can presently expect.

PREAMBLE

Some assumptions are hidden in the expression "Causes of Obesity". Why not "The Cause of Obesity"? While the cause or causes of the commonly observed large deposits of fat in humans are not well understood, there are a few distinct and diverse pathological states for which there is a limited explanation. For example, rare chronic excessive secretion of the hormones of the adrenal cortex (Cushing's syndrome) results in a characteristic abdominal adiposity. More widely distributed large deposits of fat occur in people with rare tumors of the pancreas which chronically secrete excessive amounts of the hormone insulin. In animals, analogous syndromes result from the administration of large doses of those hormones. In animals several hereditary forms of obesity occur which have been well characterized with respect to the forms of their heritability and some of the details of the mechanisms by which obesity is produced are known. In some rare instances analogous disorders have been found in humans. It is probable that the pathological mechanisms seen infrequently in human and animals are playing a role, with varying intensity, and in different combinations, in common human obesity.

Another characteristic of fat deposition in man which suggests participation of multiple and diverse mechanisms is the large range of weight of fat observed in individuals. For very lean healthy adults the amount of fat present may be as little as 9 lb (4 kg) and in very adipose persons more than 375 lb (170 kg). Not only is the total weight of fat highly variable but its regional deposition varies greatly between individuals. The two major forms of regional fat deposition are android obesity, large intra-abdominal fat deposits, and gynecoid obesity, large fat depositions principally in buttocks and legs. We should speak not of "obesity" but of "obesities".

The expression "cause" is troubling. It is entangled with the expression "necessary but not sufficient cause" and, of course, "sufficient cause". Many investigators prefer to speak of "risk factors". One fact which is clear is that coincidence is not causation. An amusing example is the observation that in New York City, during the evening, every hour on the hour the water pressure in the city lines falls. Water pressure falls when the minute hand of millions of clocks reaches the 12 o'clock mark. How do the clocks cause the water pressure to fall? Of course, they do not. The accepted explanation is that every hour on the hour the commercials appear on millions of television screens. People leave the television set and go to the bathroom, nearly simultaneously flushing millions of toilets and lowering pressure in the water lines. Another example more relevant to our present concern is that, at least in the United States, obesity, no matter how defined, is more common in African-American people. African-American people have more pigment in their skin. How does pigment in the skin cause obesity? No one believes that it does but rather some characteristic or characteristics associated with African-American people predisposes to obesity.

A useful way to think of causes is to divide them into proximate causes and ultimate causes. For example, a proximate cause might be a configuration of genes such that certain proteins are formed which participates in some way in the regulation of energy intake and output, a mechanistic formulation of immediate cause. The ultimate cause is an excess of energy intake over energy output, with storage of the excess energy as fat.

Available research in obesity strongly suggests the existence of multiple and varied proximate causes, complementary and supplementary, converging on the single ultimate cause, an excess of energy intake over energy expenditure. This relates to one of the severe difficulties encountered in studying obesity. The constellations of proximate causes are probably not the same in all people. A typical study begins by recruiting a group of people diverse for gender, age, habitual diet, and genetic characteristics. The group is divided into obese and nonobese populations and some characteristics, believed possibly to be related to proximate causes are measured. The possibility of finding clear differences is diminished by the fact that both lean and adipose populations are probably heterogeneous with respect to proximate mechanisms which regulate fat deposition. Possibly one of the reasons that the studies of the Pima Indians of Arizona have been so fruitful has been the relative homogeneity, genetically and otherwise, of that tribe. It is not certain that discoveries made in the Pimas apply to all other persons.

There is another difficulty well appreciated by researchers. Suppose that in a study comparing obese and nonobese populations, sometimes called a cross-sectional study, a difference is clearly demonstrated. Is the difference the cause of the obesity or the result of the obesity or neither? This question can be definitively answered only by a prospective study, sometimes called a longitudinal study, in which large numbers of lean people are examined, repeating the examinations years later after some of the people first studied in the lean state have become obese. In this way characteristics of those destined to become obese differ from those destined to remain lean may be discerned. Such studies are difficult to fund and difficult to execute. They require large sums of money and long intervals of time. Funding agencies need to show results as quickly as possible. Both investigators and subjects of study move on, are lost to the study.

HISTORICAL PERSPECTIVES

An association of obesity and food must have been recognized as early as the seventh century B.C. Ashurbanipal, king of ancient Assyria, reigning from 668 B.C. to 627 B.C., wrote "Does a woman conceive when a virgin or grow fat without eating?"[68].

Several centuries later Hippocrates (460 to 377) recognized a role for exercise: "Fat people who want to reduce should take their exercise on an empty stomach and sit down to their food out of breath...Thin people who want to get fat should do exactly the opposite and never take exercise on an empty stomach." He also recognized the health risks of obesity when he wrote: "Persons who are naturally very fat are apt to die earlier than those who are slender"[68].

A couple of millennia later the psychogenic hypothesis was described at book length in 1957 by Bruch who wrote "Obesity has been discussed here as an integral part of growth and development. In the face of disturbed maturation in the total personality, obesity may play a protective role, resulting in a way of life in which food and size give at least a semblance of satisfaction and security. In spite of its many obvious handicaps obesity is of positive importance in balancing an otherwise precarious life adjustment. It is a symptom, not a disease; and it cannot and should not be removed until after the underlying disturbances are corrected" [69]. This theme has been played with variations for decades and, indeed, is heard today. Cyril Connolly, English man of letters (1903-1974) wrote in the language of the man on the street: "Obesity is a mental state, a disease brought on by boredom and disappointment" [68]. An unkind point of view was presented by Gilbert Forbes in 1967 [70]. He stated: "...Fashion models are slim, children taunt their obese playmates, and doctors point out the hazards to health. What is the obese person to do under these circumstances? Eating is his prime source of satisfaction, a necessity, a means of assuaging his own frustrations, and one cannot forego that which is necessary. Denial becomes a means of coping with the actualities of a corpulent existence, for shifting the blame away from the real problem—the appetite. True, it is an immature method of dealing with reality (it is so frequently used by children), but then, many obese people are immature." The psychoanalytic vocabulary was used in a slender book by Rubin in 1970 [71]. According to this perspective, obesity is the consequence of "overeating" resulting from a "neurotic compulsion". The psychological substrate of this behavior is said to be an unconscious fear of becoming thin, which would cause anxiety, conflict and frustration in interpersonal relationships. There is an unconscious desire to be obese.

It is difficult to derive an experimentally testable hypothesis from the psychogenic formulation. However, a clear implication, expressly stated by Dr. Rubin, is that psychoanalytic treatment designed to make unconscious motivations conscious and to enhance the ability to cope with anxiety, conflict, and frustration should help obese persons to lose weight. There is no evidence, other than anecdotal, that psychoanalysis is an effective procedure for achieving weight loss [72;73].

It is important to realize that this conception imposes a heavy burden on obese persons. Not only do they suffer medical hazards and social disability but they also must bear the stigmatizing label "neurotic".

Obesity became a political issue, an aspect of the gender conflicts of the 1970s, in a basically psychoanalytic format. Orbach, consistent with Rubin, postulates an unconscious desire to become obese. She attributes obesity to "a definite and purposeful act"…, a "challenge to sex-role stereotyping and culturally defined experience of womanhood" [74]. This explanation has the same difficulties of confirmation as that of Rubin, described above, and, additionally, is disappointing in that it offers no help in understanding obesity in men. It seems incompatible with a decrease in "sex-role stereotyping" in recent decades during which there has been an increase in the prevalence of an overweight status in both men and women[4].

Does obesity predispose to mental illness, broadly defined, depression, anxiety, mood disorders, substance abuse, psychosis, neuroticism? Does mental illness predispose to obesity? Multiple cross sectional studies including thousands of people in Europe and the United States, men and women, children and adults, found no greater prevalence of major psychopathology, strictly defined and determined, in obese populations than in comparable nonobese populations [75-80]. Other cross sectional studies have found an association between obesity and mental illness, particularly mood disorders [81-83]. Cross sectional studies cannot determine whether obesity predisposes to psychiatric disorder or psychiatric disorder predisposes to obesity or both or neither. A prospective study found that mental disorder at baseline slightly predisposed to obesity during 19 years of followup [84]. It seems plausible that obesity may predispose to psychiatric disorder and psychiatric disorder may predispose to obesity.

There can be no doubt that obese persons experience obesity-related emotional distress, especially for the most obese. An Australian study of severely obese persons showed marked improvement in objective scores of psychological tests of depression following sustained surgically induced weight loss [85].

CULTURAL, PSYCHOSOCIAL, ECONOMIC AND ETHNIC FACTORS

Cultural norms can be perceived as a risk factor for obesity. In Morocco and Tunisia where "female fatness is viewed as a sign of social status and is a cultural symbol of beauty, fertility, and prosperity" the prevalence of obesity, defined by the body mass index, is hugely greater in women than men and more than 50% of women are obese by National Institute of Health guidelines [86]. However, the influence of cultural norms is not uncomplicated and not irresistible. In the United States both men and women (at least when young) express a preference for a slender body both for themselves and for the opposite gender [87]. Nevertheless for many years there has been a relentless increase in adiposity in Americans of all ages and both genders [5]. It is not easy to account for cultural preferences but their prevalence and influence have been repeatedly documented.

All over the world where the way of life of the industrialized countries has been adopted by a large segment of the population there has been a steady increase in the prevalence of obesity, specifically in the Western Hemisphere, Europe, Asia, and North Africa. Critical elements common to all these regions are believed to be a diminishing requirement for hard physical labor in earning a living, and abundant available food [13;88].

Living in an industrialized country is a major risk factor for obesity. This fact is very important. Although we cannot change our innate tendencies, we can hypothetically change our way of life. Especially in the United States we have developed a way of life which is almost exactly what one might describe if asked to design a way to produce obesity in a population. Many of us live in large far-flung suburbs, some having no sidewalks. A person seen walking in the neighborhood is regarded with suspicion. We are almost totally dependent on automobiles to get to work, to school, to stores, banks, and other service facilities. Housekeeping is aided by semi-automated machines, washers, dryers, vacuum cleaners. Our energy output is minimal. A flourish has been added to this unhealthy protocol. It has been documented that from 1977 to 1998 food portion sizes have increased substantially, especially in fast food restaurants and homes [89].

For a book-length exposition of the successful efforts of the food industry to influence the United States government public policy and recommendations see *FOOD POLITICS* by Marion Nestle [90] She documents in detail…"how the food industry uses lobbying, lawsuits, financial contributions, public relations, advertising, partnerships and alliances, philanthropy, threats, and biased information to convince Congress, federal agencies, nutrition and health professionals and the public that the science relating diet to health is so confusing that they need not worry about diets". For a book-length exposition of the very successful efforts of the food industry to induce American consumers, including children, to eat more, see *FAT LAND* by Greg Critser [91] .

Two other risk factors for obesity in the United States are poverty and membership in Native American, African-American, or Latin minorities. These factors are not easily disentangled but the association of poverty and obesity is also present in the majority Caucasian component of the population. Not only do poor adults tend to be obese but their children do also [92]. Does being poor make people obese? Does being obese make people poor? Is it the fact that neither obesity nor poverty is causative of the other but both are manifestations of some third factor responsible for both poverty and obesity? Other correlates of obesity in the majority population are female gender, marital status, income level, educational level, and rural residence [93].

Eliminating consideration of assorted confounding factors mentioned above and focusing exclusively on education and income in adults in the United States, it is abundantly clear that the fewer the years of education there have been the greater the likelihood of obesity and the lower is the income the greater is the likelihood of obesity [94]. Intuitively, many people have suggested that constraints of income and knowledge incline people to choose a diet predisposing to obesity. Some available data are supportive of this hypothesis. Critical information for support of this proposal would be: What is the diet of poor people? What does it cost in comparison with other dietary options? What are the reasons for choosing it? How might it predispose to obesity?

Although available data are not comprehensive, focused and definitive, they seem consistent with a widely held inference that low-income people in comparison with higher-income people tend to choose a diet with lower content of fresh fruits and vegetables and higher content of fats, and sugar, and of greater caloric value. Probably relevant is the demonstration that over a 15 year interval weight gain was directly associated with frequency of meals in fast food restaurants [95]. Multiple studies have shown that greater proximity to fast food relative to proximity to supermarket food is associated with obesity [96]. Energy cost, dollars/Calorie, is much lower for foods high in industrialized food, fat and sugar, than for fresh fruits and vegetables [97]. Consequently, the diet containing larger amounts of fresh fruits and vegetables recommended by nutritionists is expected to cost more than the high-fat, high-sugar diet chosen by low-income people. A large survey revealed that most Americans make dietary choices based mostly on taste and cost rather than nutritional benefits [98]. Assessing motives for human behavior in complex settings is difficult but it seems plausible that the dietary choices of low-income people result from both taste and cost factors. The idea that an *ad lib* diet with a greater fractional quantity of Calories from fats and sugar, driven by palatability and cost considerations, encourages greater caloric consumption and obesity is intuitively appealing but will be difficult to prove. Drewnowski [97] has proposed an elaboration of this idea as an "economic hypothesis" explaining the recent rapid rise in the prevalence of obesity in the industrialized world. If the hypothesis is even partially explanatory, public policy directed against obesity to be effective must offer economic and other incentives to alter the dietary choices of many people.

Christakis and Fowler have concluded on the basis of a study of social interconnections in a large population of Americans that "Network phenomena appear to be relevant to the biologic and behavioral trait of obesity, and obesity appears to spread through social ties" [99]. Given that Homo sapiens is a social mammal, as are chimpanzees and horses, it seems quite plausible that members of the herd tend to run in the same direction. The research opens a possible avenue for determination of what pushes or pulls the herd to run in a particular direction.

HEREDITY

What is a gene? When the term first appeared about one hundred years ago it designated an abstraction, a presumed unknown mechanism for the hereditary transmission of traits, properties, and characteristics. About seventy years ago it was appreciated that the production of specific proteins is a central feature of the mechanisms of heredity. The expression "one gene, one protein" became a guiding principle, but is now known to be an oversimplification. About fifty years ago the demonstration that deoxyribonucleic acid (DNA) codes the sequence of amino acid building blocks of which protein is composed initiated ongoing research revealing a system of staggering complexity in which regulation of hereditary transmission is achieved by a biochemical mechanism consisting of DNA, at least four kinds of ribonucleic acid (RNA), and innumerable proteins [100]. A contemporary definition of a gene by Snyder and Gerstein is "a complete chromosomal segment responsible for making a functional product" [101] (see **Chromosomes** in **APPENDIX 2**.)

Evidence for an important role for genes in determination of body fat is overwhelming [102]. Perhaps the simplest and at the same time most convincing evidence comes from an experimental study of male identical twins (monozygotic twins), twins genetically identical [103]. When total body fat of similar pairs of identical twins is compared, differences *within* pairs of twins are statistically significantly much less than differences *between* pairs of twins. The evidence for a strong effect of genome in this study was even more evident in comparisons of visceral adiposity. The findings were buttressed by over-feeding the subjects 1000 Calories per day for 100 days and observing the gain of total body fat and gain in visceral fat. Gains both in total body fat and in visceral adipose tissue were more similar within pairs than between pairs.

The importance of genetic influences for determination of body weight and fat, without respect to distribution of fat, is intuitively appreciated by contemplation of a variety of twin studies. A particularly convincing study was reported by Stunkard and associates [104]. Subjects were adult Swedish twins, both genders, identical twins reared together, and identical twins reared apart, fraternal twins reared together and fraternal twins reared apart. Statistically, the within pairs difference in body mass index of identical twins reared apart was almost indistinguishable from the within pairs difference of identical twins reared together. In contrast, for fraternal twins reared apart the same measures were markedly different from those of fraternal twins reared together. The authors offered a conservative conclusion: "Genetic factors appear to be major determinants of body mass index in Western society..." In the presence of identical genes environmental factors appeared to have little influence in the population studied. These results were published in 1990.

Studies of twins and numerous studies of families, not cited here, leave no possibility for doubt that heredity plays an important role in the development and maintenance of obesity. The research community has been so interested that there now exists biochemical, molecular biological evidence for the possible involvement of dozens of genes [105;106]. It seems not likely that each of those genes is involved in all instances of obesity but rather that different and smaller patterns of genes are contributing in different individuals. It seems probable that nearly every example of obesity is genetically unique but with common elements.

Very limited progress has been made in elucidating the details of genetic processes in states, such as common obesity, which are believed to have multigenic determinants. The reasons are the extreme complexity of systems apparently including gene-gene interactions, gene-environment interactions and genetic heterogeneity [12;107].

The recent rapid increase in the prevalence of obesity cannot be attributed solely to genetic factors. The genome has not changed significantly in the last generation but the environment, availability of food, absence of necessity for vigorous physical activity, has changed.

The difficulty of teasing out separate contributions of genes and environment is illustrated by a study in which it was shown that middle aged African-American women and white women with high-school-only education have similar body mass indices. However, in women with some college or college or higher as level of education increased, white women had progressively lower body mass indices. In African American women there was no decline of body mass index as educational level increased. Was the absence of a protective effect of education in African American women the consequence of a genetic effect? A suggestion has been made that educated African American women experience a psychosocial/economic milieu, different from that of their white counterparts, which predisposes to obesity [108].

There are recognized differences in the prevalence of obesity (95th percentile of Center for Disease Control and Prevention growth charts) in young children of various racial/ethnic groups. The rank order is American Indian, Hispanic, black, white, Asian [109]. Any attempt to ascribe these differences to genetics is made suspect by the difficulty of accounting for confounding socioeconomic and cultural factors.

FAT CELLS (ADIPOCYTES)

At least as early as 1953 German and Scandinavian investigators began investigating the logical idea that accumulation of body fat might result either from enlargement of fat cells, i.e. hypertrophic obesity, or increase in the number of fat cells, i.e. hyperplastic obesity, or both. Most body fat is present in the form of adipose tissue, a matrix of blood vessels, nerves and connective tissue (the substance of tendons and scars) in which several kinds of specialized cells including fat cells or adipocytes are embedded. Adipose tissue underlies the skin in most areas of the body and is found in localized accumulations in the abdomen and chest, and small deposits in various organs, muscles, liver, and kidneys.

It was soon apparent that persons with large amounts of body fat had, on average, larger fat cells than people with small or usual amounts of body fat. However, determining the number of fat cells in a person presented daunting problems. By 1969 sufficient progress had been made to allow Jules Hirsch [110] to hypothesize that overfeeding of infants during a susceptible interval in early infancy stimulates excessive multiplication of fat cells which persist throughout life and by some unknown mechanism results in accumulation of body fat. This hypothesis gave a shock of excitement to professionals who saw an opportunity to prevent obesity by regulation of the diet of infants. The hypothesis also gave a shock of guilt to parents of obese people.

When a sample of adipose tissue, obtained by surgical biopsy or by large needle aspiration, and stained for fat is viewed through a microscope it is apparent that fat occupies nearly all the volume of each of the morphologically identifiable fat cells and that in a single specimen the cells vary in size. Oculomicrometric methods can be used to determine the average size and distribution of sizes of such fat cells in a sample of adipose tissue. These methods cannot tell us how many fat cells are in the body from which the sample came.

The fact that virtually the entire volume of certain cells, characterized as fat cells or adipocytes, is occupied by fat suggested the ingenious idea of using fat as a surrogate for fat cell size and number. (see **Fat Cell Number** in **APPENDIX 1**.) Briefly, the lipid content of the average fat cell in a sample of tissue was estimated. The total body fat of the experimental subject was estimated by one of the methods described in the preceding chapter and the simple calculation of dividing the fat mass by the average fat per cell yields the estimated number of cells.

Some data were obtained which supported the Hirsch hypothesis. However, there seems to be no way confidently to estimate the number of fat cells in the body. The problem is that the average size of cells taken from different sites, abdomen, thigh, arm, buttock, or within body cavities varies significantly and unpredictably. Worse still was the recognition that enumeration of cells depended upon fat detectable by microscope in the cells. Cells containing little or no fat (preadipocytes) would not be detected. While there was no validated way to estimate the number of adipocytes in an intact human body there is available a large amount of information about the cellular mechanisms by which a preadipocytes are transformed into adipocytes. The physiological role of the transformation and its relation to obesity are not well delineated. There appears to be a maximal size which an adipocyte can attain. Consequently, in extreme obesity there may be an increase in the number of fat cells. However, this could logically be a result of obesity rather than a cause.

The Hirsch hypothesis has not been definitively disproved but it cannot be robustly supported. Echoes of the proposal are occasionally heard now but there are few adherents recently [111-114]. Many adults have participated in experiments in which they were deliberately overfed, inducing weight gain and fat deposition. Very probably there was some hyperplasia of fat depots [115]. After the experiments ended and ad lib food intake resumed these people promptly took up their usual dietary habits and their weight promptly reverted to the value with which the experiment began. It seems probable that overfed infants would also revert to some innately determined weight when overfeeding ends or would reject food in excess of that required to sustain an innately determined weight.

There have been attempts to evaluate formation of new fat cells by studying incorporation of isotopes of hydrogen (deuterium) [116] or of radioactive carbon [117] into genetic material (DNA) of fat cells isolated from humans, thus estimating the rate of proliferation of fat cells. Results have been conflicting.

In the nucleus of adipocytes and preadipocytes there has been found a protein called peroxisome proliferator activated receptor gamma 2, for convenience called PPARγ2. When this protein is bound by certain metabolites of fats or certain drugs important changes occur in the cell. In the instance of the preadipocytes the cell undergoes rapid differentiation to a mature adipocyte having the abilities to accumulate fat within itself, and to perform other characteristic metabolic and physiologic functions. In the mature adipocyte sensitivity to the actions of insulin is increased [118] The name peroxisome proliferator activated receptor is the result of the fact that a similar protein, discovered earlier, when activated by binding with certain drugs, stimulates cells of rat liver to proliferate peroxisomes which are intracellular organelles, small rounded sacs containing enzymes.

The recognition in 1994 [119] of the PPARγ2 as a regulator of adipogenesis suggested the thought that mutations of the gene mediating its synthesis might predispose to obesity (or might be a factor protective against obesity). Attempts to produce data supportive of this hypothesis have yielded mixed results. Much attention has been focused on a mutation labeled Pro12 Ala which has prevalence in some populations of about 15% [120]. There have been at least six reports of population surveys for the mutant. In a Danish population divided into lean and obese groups there was an association of the variant with higher body mass index in the obese group and in the lean group there was an association of the variant with lower BMI [121] . A German population was reported to show no association of the variant gene with obesity [122]. An American group recruited from a weight management clinic had an association of the Pro12Ala mutant with higher BMI [123]. In a Finnish study the variant gene was associated with severe obesity in women [124]. In a second Finnish study the mutation was associated with a lower BMI [125]. In Korean subjects there was no association with obesity [126]. A survey study in which dietary fat intake was assessed by questionnaire in a large population of American women reported that an observed trend toward obesity with increasing fat intake was absent in women with the mutant gene [127]. The mutated gene was protective against a diet-associated obesity.

Although study of the Pro12Ala mutant has not yielded consistent results there has been reported in four unrelated extremely obese persons the presence of a rare mutant labeled Pro115Gln. *In vitro* testing of the gene revealed enhanced adipogenic activity [128].

PREGNANCY, INFANCY, CHILDHOOD

Numerous epidemiological studies have been directed toward the hypothesis that overnutrition in pregnancy or infancy increases the risk of adult obesity. Contrariwise the hypothesis also has been advanced that under-nutrition in pregnancy or infancy increases the risk of adult obesity. The underlying rationale in both hypotheses is that the nutritional experience in utero or in infancy may "program" an individual for adult obesity. Of course, it is possible that both hypotheses are correct. They are not mutually exclusive [129]. Studies have mostly taken the form of measures of the likelihood that high birth weight (or low birth weight) increases the risk of obesity in adulthood. Results have been inconsistent [130]. A very large longitudinal study of Britons born in 1958 has shown that large birth weight has some association with adult obesity, but far more influential is large weight of mothers before pregnancy [131]. Such studies cannot distinguish between effects of genetic predisposition, and "programming" during pregnancy or infancy.

An association of low birth weight with development in adulthood of the metabolic syndrome, described in detail in Chapter Four, titled "MEDICAL HAZARDS OF OBESITY", is firmly established [132]. The syndrome is more frequent in obese persons but not confined to them. It consists of abdominal adiposity, high blood pressure, dyslipidemia, a diabetic tendency or diabetes type II (see **Diabetes Mellitus Type II**, and **Dyslipidemia** in **APPENDIX 2**.)

The epidemiological studies in humans are supported by experimental demonstrations in laboratory animals that protein-restricted diets early in pregnancy result in offspring which have reduced birth weights and in adulthood develop characteristics of the metabolic syndrome in humans [133].

In adult humans, and mice, there are marked differences in gene expression between visceral and subcutaneous fat cells and there is correlation with degree of adiposity as indexed by body mass index [134]. Does diet during pregnancy program developmental genes toward the development of the metabolic syndrome?

The idea that obese children become obese adults is seductive. It seems intuitively obvious that childhood obesity is a risk factor for adult obesity and to a significant extent this is true. It is also undoubtedly true that most obese adults were not obese children [135]. Preventing adult obesity will require measures crafted to prevent adult obesity. It is also true that most somewhat overweight children do not necessarily become overweight adults although they are significantly more likely to do so than are their lean contemporaries [136]. The likelihood of obesity at age 35 years is increased in obese older children compared with obese younger children. After about age 12 years an obese child is very likely to be obese at age 35 years [137]. A possible interpretation of these facts is that there is a subpopulation of very heavy children, especially teen-aged children, destined from early life to be heavy adults, perhaps on a genetic basis, and another subpopulation of less heavy children who experience some increased risk [138;139]. Given the difficulty of determining which obese children will experience persistence of obesity into adulthood, emphasis should be on public health measures for prevention and remediation although resolution of obesity in individual children deserves attention for prevention of development of vascular lesions and other risk factors for cardiovascular disease [140;141]. Indeed, childhood obesity is a risk factor for coronary heart disease in adulthood [142].

A perhaps related set of considerations is suggested by evidence that breastfed infants are somewhat less likely to be overweight at age 3-5 years [143] and age 9-14 years [144] than formula-fed infants. Two large meta-analyses of cohort studies (see **Cohort Studies** in **APPENDIX 2**) showed a somewhat smaller risk of later obesity for infants breast fed compared with infants formula fed [145;146]

It is important to realize the limitations of this kind of study. It proves only that mothers who choose to breast feed, for unknown reasons, are more likely to have children who years later, are less likely to be overweight, for unknown reasons. It does not prove that breast feeding protects against subsequent overweight status. That conclusion would require a trial in which there was random assignment of mother-infant pairs to breast feeding or to formula feeding, a trial not likely to be conducted. A large study of Brazilian men found no association of duration of breast feeding with obesity at age 18 years [147].

A risk factor for childhood obesity which has excited much comment is television watching. Cross sectional studies indicate a close association with childhood obesity in American children with watching 4 or more hours of television daily [148;149]. Conclusions based on cross sectional, observational studies have been confirmed by a prospective, randomized controlled study [150]. In the United States African-American children spend more hours watching television than white children. This fact has been attributed to the tendency for African-American children to live in neighborhoods in which outdoor play is unsafe.

The rising prevalence of overweight and obesity in children suggests the importance of public health measures for prevention of childhood obesity for the reason that overweight children as young as the 9 to 12 years age have been shown to have early manifestations of arterial disease [140;141]

Prolonged television watching is associated with obesity in adults as well as children. In a large prospective study of women "each two hour per day increment in TV watching was associated with a 23%…increase in obesity…" [151].

ENERGETICS

If the intake of energy into the body exceeds the expenditure of energy, there must be retained within the body a deposit of energy in some form, mostly in the form of the chemical configuration of fat:

Retained Energy = Energy Intake - Energy Expenditure

This is merely a restatement of the Law of Conservation of Energy: "Energy can be transformed but can be neither created nor destroyed." This is a fundamental law of physics which has not been seriously challenged for more than a century. Although this formulation of the ultimate cause of obesity seems obvious at this time, as recently as 1945 the medical literature offered serious discussions about it [152]. Much of the promotional effort of the commercial weight loss industry consists of denying the inescapable facts. The theme relentlessly advanced is that people can eat any desired amount if they eat what is being touted.

Recognition of the physics has been invaluable for the reason that it demands the compiling of inventories of energy intake, energy deposits and energy expenditures. Energy intake is in the form of food. Stored energy is almost entirely in the form of the chemical bonds of fat. Energy expenditure is in the form of 1) chemical work, maintenance of concentration gradients, especially of minerals, across cell membranes, the increased energy expenditure associated with assimilation of food, energy required for interconversion of some metabolic intermediates; 2) energy requirements of mechanical work, muscular contractions, including breathing and circulating blood; 3) energy expended in maintaining body temperature in an environment usually cooler than usual body temperature; and 4) energy for growth and repair of tissues.

Engineers and scientists have a great variety of ways to express quantities of energy since energy can be transformed from one mode to another. Workers in biomedicine describe energy in heat units. Again, a variety of units are available, British thermal units, Joules, Calories. In this book and most of the medical literature on this subject the unit reported is the familiar Calorie, sometimes designated as kcalories, one thousand gram-Calories. The gram-calorie is defined as the amount of heat required to increase the temperature of one gram of water from 15 degrees Celsius to 16 degrees Celsius. In some reports the unit employed is the kJoule, i.e. one thousand Joules. Joules are units of energy most typically used by physicists. One Calorie is equal to 4.18 kJoules.

Energy is taken into the body as three chemically defined components, carbohydrates, fats, and proteins. The molecules of carbohydrate, fat, and protein are made up of atoms of carbon, hydrogen, and oxygen, and, in the instance of protein, also nitrogen. Each atom is bound to one or more of the others in configurations which define the molecule as carbohydrate, fat, or protein. Formation of chemical bonds requires energy and dissolution of those bonds releases energy, some of which is manifest as heat. The remainder is transferred to energy-bearing metabolic intermediates making up the cascade of reactions terminating in the end products carbon dioxide, and water. For nitrogen the principal end products are urinary urea, ammonia, and creatinine.

Minerals, vitamins, and trace elements have so little energy value that they are not included in calculations of the energy economy. Energy-yielding components are sometimes called substrates. Typical examples of dietary carbohydrates are sugars and starches found in vegetables, fruits, sweets, and baked goods. Typical examples of dietary fats are those found in meats, butter, margarine, and vegetable oils. Important sources of dietary proteins are some beans and peas, meats, sea foods, and poultry.

In the course of devolution of energy-bearing intermediates to carbon dioxide and water, energy is expended in the formation of biosynthetic products, in mechanical work, temperature maintenance, growth and repair, and all the energy-requiring activities of living. The amounts of energy available to the body from typical substrates, carbohydrates, fats, and proteins has been determined by well-accepted physicochemical studies linked to biochemical research which has outlined the major sequences of metabolic intermediates by which carbohydrates, fats, and proteins are converted to carbon dioxide and water, with release of energy.

A detailed knowledge of foodstuffs coupled with a detailed knowledge of what someone has eaten allows for calculation of the energy produced by metabolism of the diet. Metabolism of 1 gram of typical carbohydrate provides 3.74 Calories; for one gram of typical fat the value is 9.46 Calories, and for typical protein is 4.32 Calories.

In some research concerning the metabolism of obese people, in which dietary composition is critical, diets are assayed and dispensed to the experimental subjects. It has been repeatedly demonstrated that many obese people self-reporting their diets consistently under-report their consumption [153;154] This does not mean that obese people as a group are less truthful than their lean neighbors. It seems that obese people have a selective unawareness of their food intake and this is probably a part of the syndrome of obesity.

The inventory of components of energy expenditure which has been the subject of important research is summarized in the table below: Percentage daily energy expenditure values shown are typical and may not apply to an individual at a particular time.

Component	% Daily Energy Expenditure
Resting metabolic rate	60
Thermogenic effect of food	10
Spontaneous physical activity	10
Voluntary physical activity	20

Total daily energy expenditure can be estimated in free-living persons by a procedure called "Doubly Labeled Water". The principles of the doubly labeled water procedure are outlined in **APPENDIX 1**.

Water, labeled with nonradioactive isotopes is administered to the subject and samples of urine are collected for isotopic analysis during the interval over which the energy expenditure is measured. The values obtained are Calories per unit time, usually Calories per day, during which the subject is free-living and has customary activity. Measurements by the doubly labeled water method require expensive equipment and advanced skills and are not widely available.

The resting metabolic rate, sometimes called the basal metabolic rate, is the rate of expenditure of energy by a person resting quietly in bed in the morning at comfortable ambient temperature, having eaten nothing since midnight (fasting). During and following a meal there is an increase in the metabolic rate, an addition to the resting energy expenditure, of variable quantity and duration. It is called the thermogenic effect of food and has been thought to be the energy cost of absorption and assimilation of food. Some details concerning this component are discussed below. In estimating resting metabolic rate and the thermogenic effect of food, subjects are asked to avoid spontaneous physical activity, "fidgeting", which is a small but variable element in the total energy economy. Spontaneous physical activity consists of a myriad of movements of extremities and head occurring largely unconsciously and serving no outwardly directed purpose although they must satisfy some inner need.

Several combinations of components of the inventory are possible. The total daily expenditure of energy can be measured by doubly labeled water. The resting metabolic rate and the thermic effect of food can be estimated by indirect calorimetry. The difference between the doubly labeled water value and the sum of resting metabolic rate plus energy expenditure of spontaneous physical activity plus the thermogenic effect of food, measured in a whole body indirect calorimeter, is the daily energy expenditure for physical activity.

The resting metabolic rate is measured by indirect calorimetry, a procedure in which the carbon dioxide added to expired air, and the oxygen removed from inspired air are measured. The ratio, (rate of expiration of carbon dioxide)/(rate of consumption of oxygen), together with the rate of urinary excretion of nitrogenous compounds permits calculation of the rate of consumption (oxidation, "burning") of the substrates carbohydrate, fat, and protein separately. The ratio of carbon dioxide added to oxygen removed, measured in the respired air, is called the respiratory quotient *(RQ)*, an important term in the equations used for calculation of differential substrate oxidation (see **Indirect Calorimetry** in **APPENDIX 1**)

The resting metabolic rate which some contemporary laboratory researchers sometimes call the basal metabolic rate should not be confused with a now obsolete procedure, the "basal metabolism test", usually performed in a physician's office. The purpose was to aid in the diagnosis of thyroid disease. It was subject to an array of serious errors and there are now better approaches to the diagnosis of thyroid disease. It is now seldom performed.

Prospective studies probing for metabolic predictors of weight gain, of obesity, have focused on resting metabolic rate, on energy expenditure consequent to physical activity, and on the rate of fat oxidation.

As early as 1922 there were efforts to probe the nature of obesity by analysis of respiratory gases, indirect calorimetry [155]. Early efforts were not fruitful for many reasons. The necessity to distinguish between causes of obesity and consequences of obesity was not recognized. There were technical problems in accurate measurements of respiratory gases and setting the conditions for conduct of the procedure. The more sophisticated mathematical, statistical, procedures now known to be needed for adequate analysis of results were not in wide use. The latter difficulty relates to the fact that it was appreciated that large people, obese or not, would be expected to have higher metabolic rates than small people. Early investigators attempted to deal with this difficulty by computing a ratio of metabolic rate to body surface area, the latter calculated by equations of necessarily approximate accuracy. Gender and age specific allowances were made. This is intuitively appealing since heat loss is related to surface area. However, it was not very useful. More recently it has come to be understood that the resting metabolic rate is closely correlated to indices of metabolically active tissue. Indices used have been the fat-free mass estimated by skin fold thickness, by total body potassium, by hydrodensitometry, by isotopic measurements of total body water and the lean body mass derived from dual-energy x-ray absorptiometry. These techniques, described in the preceding chapter, were not available to early investigators.

A fundamental, inescapable difficulty in studying the energetics of obesity is the consequence of the fact that very small daily differences in energy expenditure or energy intake, difficult to measure, can over periods of months or years result in very large weight gains or losses. Assume, on the basis of many physiological data, that:

One pound (0.45 kg) of weight gained requires 3500 Calories; and
Average efficiency of excess energy conservation in the form of weight gain is 50%.

It can be calculated that a daily excess of energy intake over energy expenditure of 100 Calories per day, resulting from the daily ingestion of two pats of butter (14 Grams of fat), will result in one year in a weight gain of 5.2 pounds (2.3 Kilograms).

The status of a low resting metabolic rate as a risk factor for future obesity is controversial. In 1988 Ravussin and coworkers [156] reported a study of 126 adult Pima Indians of Arizona (men and women) in which they found that a relatively low resting metabolic rate enhanced the probability of marked weight gain during a follow up period of up to four years. Subsequently at least three other groups of investigators have reported data from prospective investigations which might have been expected to support a finding of low resting metabolism as a predictor of obesity but did not. In one study the subjects were middle aged men, [154] in another infants [157] and, in the third, subjects were postmenopausal women who had lost weight and regained it over a period of four years. In the latter study women who were normal weight and had never been obese were compared with women who had been obese but had reduced to normal weight. The comparison was repeated four years later after the formerly obese women had regained most of the weight lost. No relationship was found between the amount of weight regained and the resting metabolic rate in the reduced state. No difference was found in the resting metabolic rate of women reduced to normal weight and the comparison lean never-obese group [158;159]. Possibly a low resting metabolic rate is a precursor of weight gain in Pima Indians but not frequently in other populations, or possibly these conflicts of data, like so many others in science, are not fully explainable at this time. Some support for the idea that resting metabolic metabolism is reduced in some racial groups, predisposing to obesity, is found in a cross-sectional study demonstrating that lean pubertal African-American girls have a lower resting metabolic rate than a matched control group of Caucasian girls [160]. Both Pima Indians and female African-Americans are notoriously at risk for obesity. The topic is important because resting metabolic rate is usually more than one-half the total daily energy expenditure. A small fractional difference, difficult to detect, could represent a large absolute difference which in sufficient time could be the source of obesity, only if energy intake exceeded energy expenditure.

The twenty-four hour energy expenditure seems somewhat better established than the resting metabolic rate as a risk factor for weight gain. Investigators of the Pima Indians have again been prominent. They built an indirect calorimeter in the form of a room large enough to permit activities of daily living. It is equipped with flow meters, temperature controls, and sensors for oxygen and carbon dioxide and allows for sleeping, eating, toileting, bathing and television watching for one or more whole days during which energy expenditure is continuously monitored. Ravussin and colleagues [156] found, in a prospective study that persons with a relatively low rate of twenty four hour energy expenditure, statistically adjusted for fat mass, fat-free mass, age, and gender have a four-fold increased risk of gaining 16.6 lb. (7.5 kg) during two years. A relatively low twenty-four hour energy expenditure rate may be present as a risk factor early in life. Roberts and collaborators [157] reported that infants who became obese at one year of age had a 20.7% lower twenty-four hour expenditure at age three months than infants not becoming obese at one year. Energy expenditure was measured by the doubly-labeled water technique in children living freely at home with their mothers. Comparisons were of children becoming obese and born to obese mothers with children not becoming obese and born to both lean and obese mothers.

If twenty-four hour energy expenditure is lower in persons destined to become obese, which component or components are low? As described above, an association of low basal, resting metabolic energy expenditure with obesity is controversial. In 1976 Pittet and colleagues [161], in a cross-sectional study, reported that the thermogenic effect of glucose is lower in obese persons. Subsequently a variety of investigations were performed in which serious difficulties were recognized. The thermogenic effect of food is the most variable component in typical indirect calorimetry studies. The timing of the beginning and end are often uncertain. It is not clear how the results should be expressed e.g. as a fraction of the caloric value of the food ingested, as heat per square meter of surface area, or per unit weight of fat-free mass [162]. The definitive study seems to have been accomplished by Tataranni [163] who found in a prospective study with average 2.9 years follow up of Pima Indians that thermogenic effect of food expressed in three different ways is not a risk factor for subsequent obesity. Conflicting findings by respected investigators may be the consequence of heterogeneity in and between populations studied.

It is well established that there are large individual differences in the tendency to deposit fat and gain weight in response to the same amount of overfeeding [103]. Many different explanations are more or less plausible. This line of thought suggested an interesting prospective study, reported in 1999, by Levine and associates [164]. They measured twenty-four hour energy expenditure by the doubly labeled water technique in nonobese people taking weight-maintaining diets. They then overfed the people diets containing 1000 Calories per day in excess of their individual weight-maintaining diets for 8 weeks. Average weight gain was 10.4 lb. (4.7 kg) and the range was an astonishing 3.1 lb. (1.4 kg) to 16 lb. (7.2 kg). Fat gain, measured by dual energy x-ray absorptiometry, ranged from 0.8 lb. (0.36 kg) to 9.4 lb. (4.23kg). Resting metabolic rate and thermogenic effect of eating were estimated by indirect calorimetry before and after weight gain. During the 8 weeks of overfeeding the subjects were free-living and were monitored. It was insisted that they avoid any form of physical activity except their usual activities of daily living. Specifically, exercise for sports and fitness-related activities, which the investigators called volitional activity, was forbidden. The sum of resting metabolism and thermogenic effect of food, measured by indirect calorimetry, was subtracted from the 24 hour total energy expenditure, measured by the doubly labeled water procedure, to obtain what was called the "nonexercise activity thermogenesis". As in previously published reports of overfeeding experiments, average resting metabolic rate and average thermogenic effect of eating of the group increased but neither was quantitatively related to the amount of fat deposited. Nonexercise activity thermogenesis was closely negatively related to weight gain and fat deposition.

The authors defined nonexercise activity thermogenesis as "thermogenesis that accompanies physical activities other than volitional exercise, such as the activities of daily living, fidgeting, spontaneous muscle contraction, and maintaining posture when not recumbent". In their experiment they did not look specifically for the presence or absence of "physical activities other than volitional exercise" and do not suggest a mechanism by which increased dietary intake might increase it.

In subsequent experiments Levine and associates [165] have attached arrays of motion and position sensors to free-living subjects, both lean and obese, both genders, and measured total energy expenditure (doubly labeled water), energy expenditure walking, standing, sitting (indirect calorimetry) in addition to the thermic effect of food and the basal metabolic rate. Obese subjects were sitting an average164 minutes per day more than lean subjects. Lean persons were standing 152 minutes per day more than obese persons. If the obese people had practiced the same postural distribution as the lean people they would have expended an estimated average additional 352 Calories per day. Did the obese subjects sit more because they were heavier or were they heavier, at least partly, because they sat more? To answer this question, for 10 days the lean group was overfed, gaining 4 kg (8.9 pounds), and the obese subjects were underfed, losing 8 kg (17.6 pounds). The distribution of sitting/standing time remained the same as before the loss and gain of weight. The authors suggested that allocation of time of posture is "biologically determined".

An effect of nonexercise activity thermogenesis, in the sense postulated by Levine et al., was documented in a 1992 study of Pima Indians [166] in which a room-sized indirect calorimeter was fitted with radar-based motion detectors allowing estimation of the percentage of time the subject had detectable movement during 24 hours. The investigators called this value an index of "spontaneous physical activity", which they thought was mostly "fidgeting". Among males only, during followup averaging 33 months, spontaneous physical activity was negatively correlated with the rate of fat mass increase, determined by hydrodensitometry. The tendency toward increased spontaneous physical activity had a familial distribution and the authors concluded that "spontaneous physical activity is a familial trait that may play a role in the pathogenesis of obesity".

A very large body of knowledge exists concerning metabolic processes in which the energy of food is converted to heat and to intermediate substances which provide energy for chemical and mechanical work and for energy storage. There is also a body of knowledge concerning metabolic processes in which the energy of food is converted to heat only, without production of energy-rich intermediate substances capable of fueling work or storage of energy. Such processes are called "uncoupled" for the reason that the metabolic transformation of ingested food energy is not coupled to production of chemical or other work or energy storage through the production of intermediate energy-rich substances. Several genes mediate the production of several different proteins possibly capable of inducing uncoupling under defined circumstances. Efforts to associate mutations of these genes with obesity in humans have not been successful.

In 2009 there were published three independent demonstrations of the presence of brown adipose tissue in adult humans [167-169], achieved by use of the modern imaging technology positron emission tomography (PET scanning). Two kinds of adipose tissue have been recognized: white adipose tissue, commonly found under the skin and in intraabdominal deposits and brown adipose tissue, found in the neck and upper anterior chest in some adult humans. Until recently it was generally believed that brown adipose tissue is present and physiologically important in rodents and in human infants but absent from human adults. (It is brown as a consequence of containing some iron compounds). It has been shown to be important in regulation of body temperature and regulation of energy balance in rodents. Its effects are achieved by "uncoupling" of metabolism of brown fat cells, increased metabolic rate, oxidation of fat to carbon dioxide and water producing heat but no energy-rich intermediates used for physiological work or storage.

In adult humans brown adipose tissue has been shown to be activated by cold exposure, as in rodents, and to be reduced in quantity in overweight and obese persons. The quantity is positively correlated with resting metabolic rate. There is a large, detailed literature concerning the properties of brown adipose tissue in rodents which has been ably reviewed by Cannon and Nedergaard [170]. If similar characteristics are shown to be present in adult humans it will improve our understanding of several findings.

The observation that some individuals deposit large amounts of body fat while ingesting increased caloric intake while other persons gain little or no increased body fat has led to speculations that the differences may be attributable to individual differences in diet-induced thermogenesis, sometimes called adaptive thermogenesis, or facultative thermogenesis.

In both mice and men sustained exposure to cold or to sustained dietary caloric excess induces sustained increased metabolic rate, as Levine and associates and others have reported. The response to diet has been called diet-induced thermogenesis. Ingestion of a diet of caloric value in excess of that required for maintenance of usual body weight and usual physical activity (overfeeding) results in increased resting metabolic rate and, in mice, increased activity of brown adipose tissue. On the other hand, in mice and men, underfeeding (ingestion of a diet calorically insufficient to maintain usual body weight with usual physical activity) results in a reduced resting metabolic rate [159;171]. In mice, fasting or food restriction results in inactivation and atrophy of brown adipose tissue.

In mice it has been shown that genetic modifications which abolish the capacity of cells to respond to the neurohormones of the peripheral sympathetic nervous system abolish diet-induced thermogenesis and induce obesity [172]. Brown adipose tissue in mice is entirely under control of the sympathetic nervous system. A possible role for the sympathetic nervous system in producing human obesity has been provided by prospective study of Pima Indians in which it was demonstrated that reduced secretion of sympathetic neurohormones predicts weight gain [173], possibly as a result of reduced diet-induced thermogenesis.

Possible sympathetic nervous system effects, uncoupling effects, and fidgeting are not mutually exclusive causes contributing to obesity.

As early as 1940 there were reports of cross-sectional studies comparing physical activity of obese and nonobese children and, subsequently, adults. They were unanimous in concluding that obese persons are less physically active than lean persons. Of course, such investigations could not distinguish between the causes of obesity and the results of obesity. Now we have appropriate prospective, longitudinal, data. Many students of this subject now think of physical inactivity as a risk factor for obesity important as or more important than any other [174]. Emphasis on physical inactivity as an important risk factor is supported by data showing that during the early years, beginning about 1980, that the prevalence of obesity rose rapidly while caloric intake may have stabilized or diminished at least in some communities in the United States [175] and Britain [7]. Equally importantly, it seems that increasing nonexercise activity could be a major defense against obesity.

The human gastrointestinal tract contains a vast number of microorganisms with tens of thousands of species represented. The mixture of species of organisms found in the intestines of obese persons differs from that found in lean persons. Diet- mediated weight loss by obese persons results in changes in the spectrum of intestinal microbes [176]. Experiments in mice demonstrate that animals with intestinal microbes usual for mice have more body fat than similar germ-free mice with the same food intake and the difference results from a more efficient harvest of ingested dietary substances, especially fiber, nondigestible carbohydrate of plant origin [177].

Does the composition of the intestinal microflora play a causative role in obesity or is it the consequence of obesity? A causative role is suggested by a report that children destined to be overweight at age 7 have an intestinal flora in infancy different from that of contemporaries destined to be lean at age 7. Altered intestinal flora preceded overweight status [178]. Twin studies indicate that host genetics influences the composition of the intestinal microflora [179;180].

It is possible that ongoing research will reveal an effective method of treating obesity by manipulating the gut bacterial flora [181].

The recent recognition of the importance of physical exercise in prevention of obesity has stimulated suggestions for social and community programs to enhance physical activity, walking paths, bicycling paths, swimming pools, and higher density housing to discourage use of automobiles [182].

No matter what the rate of energy expenditure, obesity can occur only if a rate of energy intake sufficient to permit energy storage is sustained. Regulation of body fat stores implies regulation not only of energy expenditure but regulation of energy intake.

METABOLISM, BIOCHEMISTRY

Another risk factor for obesity was delineated in a study of Pima Indians reported in 1990 [183]. It was a prospective, i.e. longitudinal, study of 111 subjects in which indirect calorimetry revealed a relatively greater ratio of carbohydrate oxidation to fat oxidation in subjects destined to gain weight. Statistical means were employed to adjust for body composition, (measured by densitometry) age, gender, and immediately prior weight gain or loss. All subjects were taking a standardized conventional diet, (50% carbohydrate, 30% fat, 20% protein) the caloric value of which was adjusted to maintain the weight of each individual. In subsequent followup for three years subjects with the highest ratio of carbohydrate to fat oxidation were 2.5 times as likely to gain at least 11 pounds (5 kg) as those with the lowest ratio. These results were confirmed in 1992 in a study of 775 Caucasian men of middle to upper socioeconomic standing [154].

This metabolic characteristic may be, quantitatively, an important contributing cause of obesity and it fits with satisfying elegance what has been learned subsequently about the metabolism of fat, carbohydrate and protein. Fat metabolism is different from that of carbohydrate and protein. Carbohydrate is not converted to important quantities of fat in humans taking any likely diet. Not long ago students of metabolism assumed there must be significant conversion of carbohydrate to fat, called *de novo* lipogenesis. That belief was based on readily induced conversion of carbohydrate to fat in laboratory rats and mice. However, several lines of evidence, most convincingly radioisotopic studies, indicate that average *de novo* lipogenesis in humans taking any sustainable diet is small, [116;184;185]. However, there is large interindividual variability. Perhaps future research may yield some significant findings for individuals. To the small extent that average *de novo* lipogenesis occurs it seems to occur equally in overfed lean and obese people [186].

If a calorically sufficient mixed diet is abruptly supplemented with a large amount of carbohydrate, fat oxidation is suppressed and whatever fat is in the diet tends to be stored and weight is gained in succeeding days. The rate of carbohydrate oxidation attains the rate of carbohydrate ingestion in hours or days. If a calorically sufficient mixed diet is abruptly supplemented by a large amount of fat, there is virtually no effect on the rate of fat oxidation and the excess fat is almost all stored as body fat in succeeding days. These metabolic effects probably are mediated by insulin, a hormone secreted by the pancreas which is essential for the normal metabolism of carbohydrates (see **Insulin** in **APPENDIX 2**).

These observations of the gross metabolic characteristics of people are nicely supplemented and extended by biochemical studies. Within cells of liver and muscle, especially, there is found an enzyme (a protein catalyst) which directs fatty components of diet and metabolism either to a pathway resulting in oxidation ("burning") or to a pathway resulting in storage in fat cells. The enzyme has the awkward name carnitine palmitoyltransferase I and is understandably often designated CPTI. Its activity enhances fat oxidation. Its inhibition results in directing fat metabolism toward fat deposition. The enzyme is inhibited by a product of the metabolism of carbohydrates, called malonyl-CoA. CPT activity is lower in muscles of obese people who also manifest reduced oxidation of fat [187-190]. Weight loss in obese persons by dietary restriction increased fat oxidation by muscle little [190] or not at all [189], indicating that the defect is not caused by obesity and may contribute to the development of obesity. Exercise and fasting increase activity of the enzyme as a result of increased consumption of malonyl-CoA and thereby reduction of concentration of malonyl-CoA. Subsequently fat oxidation by muscle increases. Inactivity allows accumulation of malonyl-CoA, inhibition of CPTI and reduced oxidation of fat by muscle [191].

Intuitively, it might be expected that mutations resulting in deficient CPTI activity would result in obesity. The observed facts are complex. CPTI enzymatic activity has been associated with three different proteins encoded by three different genes. One protein is found in liver (CPTIA), another in muscle (CPTIB) and a third in brain (CPT1C). Mutation of only the liver enzyme has been recognized in humans [192]. Mutation of the liver CPTI gene has been frequently lethal. In case reports, first symptoms have typically appeared in infancy or childhood during fasting or viral illness. Observations have included low blood glucose concentrations, sometimes resulting in irreversible brain damage or death, and biochemical evidence in blood and urine of diminished oxidation of fat [193;194]. Adaptation to fasting is critically dependent on oxidation of fat in liver. Obese people do adapt to fasting. These findings suggest that the reduced activity of CPTI in obese people is not the consequence of a frequent mutation of the gene encoding the protein but is the result of regulation in which fat deposition is enhanced which may or may not be attributable to a gene, other than the gene for CPTI.

However, incremental fat storage, no matter how mediated, obviously cannot continue indefinitely and it does not. During an interval of weeks or months, as fat stores gradually attain a definite quantity, different for individuals, the rate of fat oxidation increases, eventually attaining the rate of ingestion, and a new steady state for body weight, quantity of stored fat, and rate of fat oxidation ensues [195;196]. Although documented in less detail, it seems that a calorically insufficient diet of any composition results in a rate of oxidation of fat in excess of the rate of fat ingestion and fat loss occurs until a diminishing mass of fat brings the rate of fat oxidation to the rate of fat ingestion.

The result is that for people taking mixed diets, fat mass is determined by caloric balance (energy intake minus energy expenditure) and some mechanism which individually adjusts fat mass and fat oxidation. When diet is calorically sufficient, fat mass is that which, individually innately determined, allows fat oxidation to equal fat ingestion. We would expect this system to generate a relatively stable fat mass and body weight despite day-to-day changes in the caloric value and composition of the diet. It seems to do so but with large differences of fat mass between individuals. Important questions for which there are no completely satisfying answers are: What determines energy intake, other than availability? What determines energy expenditure, other than necessity for physical activity and the maintenance of body functions? What couples the rate of fat oxidation to fat mass? What determines the amount of fat mass which will be associated with a rate of fat oxidation equal to the rate of fat intake?

ENDOCRINOLOGY

A generally held belief, based more on incidental observation than on published systematic data, is that body weight tends to be very consistent day to day. Reductions occurring as a consequence of illness or dieting are rapidly restored with recovery from illness or cessation of dieting. Constancy of weight almost requires constancy of fat mass. Apparent day-to-day stability of the fat mass has stimulated discussion of an individual "set point" for fat mass analogous to the set point for temperature regulated by the thermostat in a building. This concept implies the existence of a sensor or sensors of fat mass and also an effector or effectors increasing or decreasing fat mass with feedback loops stabilizing fat mass. Until 1994 no clear cut mechanism having these properties was known. In that year the gene mediating synthesis of a protein subsequently called leptin (Greek for thin) was isolated and sequenced.

For full comprehension of the role of leptin and some subsequent topics it is necessary to understand some basic concepts of endocrinology, traditionally defined as the study of the glands of internal secretion, and their secretions which mediate functions at a distance from the gland of origin. The traditional glands of internal secretion are the anterior pituitary, posterior pituitary, testis, ovary, thyroid, parathyroid, adrenal cortex, adrenal medulla, and pancreas. A "hormone" in the traditional sense is a substance produced in a "gland" and secreted into the blood, which takes it to other cells, tissues or organs where it mediates a change in the state or activities of the target cells, tissues, or organs. The quantity of hormone secreted, in weight units, is usually very small and has no significant energy value. A well known example is insulin, a deficiency of which is the cause of diabetes mellitus type I (see **Diabetes** in **APPENDIX 2**.) Insulin is secreted by certain cells of the intra-abdominal gland called the pancreas. It is carried in the blood to all cells, tissues, and organs of the body. Some of the best known actions of insulin are on muscle, liver, and adipose tissue. In muscle the uptake of glucose ("animal sugar") from blood is accelerated by exposure to insulin and in liver the conversion of glycogen ("animal starch") to glucose, with subsequent release into blood, is suppressed. The result is a decline in the concentration of glucose in the blood. In adipose tissue an effect of insulin is to reduce the rate of conversion of intracellular fat, triglyceride, to glycerol and fatty acids and their subsequent release into the blood stream.

This tidy traditional picture was disrupted by the recognition during the last half century that substances having the general characteristics of hormones may be secreted by cells which are not part of a gland, in the usual sense. Leptin is an example. The most important source is the fat cells, adipocytes, scattered through the body, clearly not a gland, in the usual sense. It has long been recognized that the distance from its cell of origin at which a hormone acts need not be very great. The effect could be on a nearby cell or, indeed, on an adjacent cell, in which instance the effect is not called an endocrine effect but is called a paracrine effect. The secretions of neurons, neurohormones, by which one neuron signals an adjacent neuron, could be considered paracrine secretions.

Before a hormone can exert its characteristic action it must bind to a receptor, a relatively hormone-specific protein found in or on the target cell, and synthesized by the target cell under control of its genes. The receptor is said to be "activated" by binding with the hormone and there follows a sequence of events resulting in a characteristic alteration of activities or states of the target cell.

This conception of a far-from-simple process has in recent years been made more complex by the discovery of proteins having the characteristics of receptors, including binding-activation by typical hormones, which are also bound and activated by products of metabolism, rather than hormones. An example, discussed below is the peroxisome proliferator activated receptor family at least some of which are bound and activated by fatty acids, components of lipid metabolism.

Obviously there is a blurring of definitions and concepts, endocrine, metabolic, and hormonal. This is important because, to quote a wise admonition, "if you don't talk right you can't think right". A solution to this problem could be abandonment of the traditional terminology and to speak and think of integrative systems and subsystems, with components of organs, tissues, cells, and intracellular organelles interrelated by molecular signals. Completely adopting such language would be a reach for most of us. Consequently I will use the older terminology where it seems appropriate.

The history of discovery of leptin and the subsequent explosion of penetrating research is fascinating and reveals much about modern science. In 1950 Ingalls and collaborators [197] described a mutant strain of obese mice. Subsequently the strain was bred, and maintained, and characterized by Coleman and Hummel. Details were provided in a series of papers published from 1967 to 1975 [198]. The animals were obese, inactive, and sexually immature, had diabetes, resembling that associated with obesity in humans, type II diabetes mellitus, and ate ravenously. The mutant animals were made subjects of a series of parabiosis experiments. Parabiosis is a state in which lateral tissues of two animals are surgically fused to produce the functional equivalent of Siamese twins. Blood from each animal circulates in the blood vessels of the other. The two creatures have, to an extent, a common circulation. When a mutant obese diabetic mouse was parabiosed with a normal mouse, there were no metabolic changes in the normal animal but the metabolism of the mutant animal was improved. It ate less, lost weight and its diabetes was ameliorated. The authors concluded that the normal mouse, but not the mutant mouse, produces a "satiety factor" secreted into the common blood stream.

Subsequently a significant literature characterizing rodent obesity has developed and has had important applications to human physiology. There have also been impressive gains in the technology of molecular biology, the study of genetics, cellular physiology, and protein chemistry. In 1994 Zhang and collaborators [199] announced the isolation and characterization of a gene responsible for the "satiety factor" in mice, and its human homologue. Subsequently a second strain of mice with a different mutation in the same gene has been identified [200]. The availability of the gene has made it possible to produce, by the methods of recombinant DNA technology (see **APPENDIX 2.**) useful quantities of the "satiety factor", now called leptin [201]. The chemistry and many of the biological properties of leptin, a protein, have been undergoing rapid delineation in an explosion of research.

When normal mouse leptin is injected into mutant mice, in which the gene required to produce leptin is mutant (defective) and whose blood contains no active leptin, they reduce their food intake, increase their energy expenditure, become more active, and lose weight. Nearly all of the weight lost is fat.

It was initially hoped that much human obesity would be similar to that in the mutant mice, a deficiency of leptin. This appealing idea was quite immediately disproved by the finding that people with "ordinary obesity" had greater than normal concentrations of leptin in their blood.

Disproof of the simple and attractive hypothesis that "ordinary obesity" is leptin-deficiency does not imply that leptin has no role in the normal regulation of body fat deposits in man for, indeed, it seems to have a very important set of functions. Perhaps the simplest and most convincing evidence comes from a study of two children, cousins in a highly consanguineous family [202]. Both children had normal birth weights and neither parent was obese. Both children gained weight rapidly immediately after birth and were said to be constantly hungry though they ate more than their siblings of normal weight. Leptin was almost absent from their blood. Sequencing and characterization of the gene mediating leptin synthesis revealed the same mutation of the leptin gene in both children. At the time of publication of the first report they were aged 8 years and 2 years and consequently little could be known of their growth and development to adulthood. However, they seemed, so far as could be determined, to experience pathology similar to that in the mice.

At age 9 years the older of these children was subjected to a one year course of leptin therapy, given by daily injection in doses estimated to provide a concentration of leptin in blood of 10% of normal, calculated on the basis of age, gender, and body composition. Fat mass and fat-free mass were estimated by dual energy X-ray absorptiometry. Diet and activity were ad lib. She began immediately to lose weight, reduced her food intake, and increased her physical activity. Weight loss was almost entirely fat. Total daily energy expenditure estimated by the doubly labeled water technique showed a persistent energy deficit attributable almost entirely to reduced food intake [203].

Three additional persons have been found who had a mutation of the leptin gene, one adult male, one adult female and a female child, aged 6 years. All were very obese, and the two adults showed failure of development of the reproductive tract.

It is gratifying to record that a subsequent report by the above authors, and others, details beneficial effects of treatment of the three children mentioned above for periods of 10 to 50 months. All lost weight, almost entirely as fat mass despite an expected growth of lean body mass, measured by dual X-ray absorptiometry. Loss of fat was almost entirely the consequence of reduced *ad libitum* food intake. Basal metabolic rates, adjusted for lean body mass, measured by indirect calorimetry, and free-living total energy expenditure, adjusted for lean body mass, measured by the doubly labeled water technique, showed no consistent changes. The oldest child was prepubertal and underwent an apparently normal puberty during treatment [204]. Remedying leptin deficiency made these children apparently normal.

In both mice and men, leptin is almost entirely a secretion of fat cells (adipocytes). Consequently, the more adipose is an individual, the greater is the amount of leptin produced, and the higher is the concentration of leptin in blood. Under most circumstances concentrations of leptin in blood of women are greater than those of men. This does not seem surprising since women typically have a higher proportion of fat in their body composition. However, studies of leptin production by excised fatty tissue show more leptin production per unit weight of fat cells from women than from men. This appears to be the result of a stimulatory effect of female hormones (estrogens) on leptin production, and, perhaps, an inhibiting effect of male hormones (androgens). A third influence contributing somewhat to the relatively higher concentration of leptin in the blood of women is the gender differential of fat distribution. As we all know, men tend to have protuberant abdomens, reflecting the presence of intra-abdominal fat, and women tend to have relatively larger buttocks and thighs, reflecting the presence of fat under the skin. Fatty tissue excised from subcutaneous depots secretes more leptin than a similar amount of fatty tissue excised from intra-abdominal depots of the same individual, irrespective of gender [205].

Conceptions of the manner in which leptin influences the amount of fat deposition in humans have been shaped by experiments in mice of a sort which could not be performed in humans. Injections of leptin into the brain and into peripheral blood vessels of normal mice, or mutant leptin-deficient mice or mice genetically modified to be unable to produce certain neurohumors which influence feeding behaviors have resulted in the broad outline of a highly redundant system in which leptin plays a central role in regulating body fat. At certain sites in the brain leptin binds to its receptors resulting in stimulation of production of neurohormones, paracrine hormones produced by neurons, which influence a sequence of downstream neurons which mediate inhibition of feeding (α-melanocyte stimulating hormone) and also mediate inhibition of production of neurohormones which by neural mechanisms enhance feeding (neuropeptide Y, agouti-related-protein, melanin concentrating hormone, orexins). The neurohormones are chemical messengers, substances released by one neuron which stimulate a neuron downstream in the circuitry. The location and some of the functional characteristics of downstream structures are known or suspected as a result of brain-lesioning or stimulation experiments in rats begun fifty years before the discovery of leptin.

The fact that the names of some of the foregoing neurohormonal inhibitors and stimulators of feeding seem unrelated to control of fat deposition is the result of the fact that these substances have long been known and studied for physiological activities not directly related to leptin. This eventual recognition of previously unknown properties of these substances is characteristic of science which is like the miser who saves left-overs on bottle caps—nothing is wasted, everything is used—eventually.

Figure 1 is a schematic representation of present conceptions of the role of leptin in the regulation of body fat. The figure represents a pair of linked conventional negative feedback loops familiar to all engineers and biomedical scientists. The right side of the figure indicates that increased fat and consequent increased secretion of leptin mediate neural signals in the central nervous system which bring about reduced food-seeking behavior and increased metabolic rate. The consequence is inhibited fat accumulation and reduced leptin production. Contrariwise, on the left side of the figure reduced fat stores, with reduced leptin secretion activates neural signals which result in increased food-seeking and reduced metabolic rate. Fat accumulation is then increased.

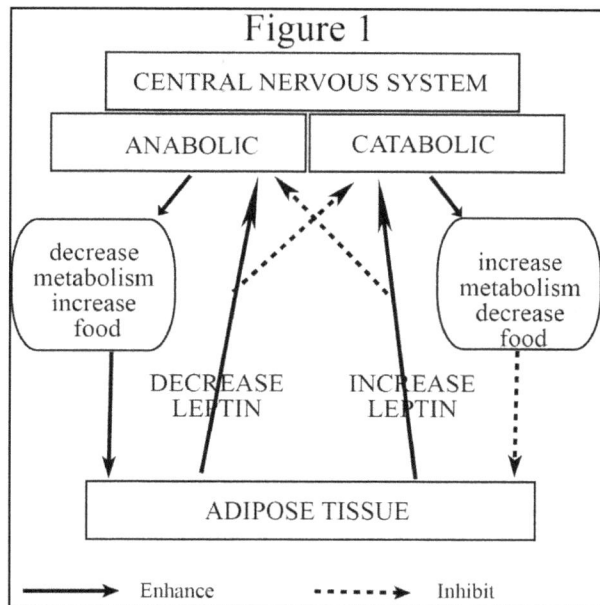

Figure 1

CENTRAL NERVOUS SYSTEM

ANABOLIC   CATABOLIC

decrease metabolism increase food

increase metabolism decrease food

DECREASE LEPTIN   INCREASE LEPTIN

ADIPOSE TISSUE

→ Enhance   ·····▶ Inhibit

On the basis of Figure 1, one might suspect that a mutation of the gene directing synthesis of the brain receptor for leptin would result in people very similar to people in which a mutation of the gene directing synthesis of leptin results in failure to synthesize leptin. Indeed, several such people have been described [206].

In addition to its effects on the central nervous system, leptin has a direct effect on muscle. It activates a muscle enzyme called 5'-AMP-activated protein kinase (AMPK) which inhibits another enzyme, acetyl coenzyme A carboxylase (ACC). ACC enhances fat synthesis and, therefore, its inhibition limits fat accumulation in muscle [207].

This is a complex system and the diagram above presents a simplified conception. Much work remains to be done. However, it is clear that people with "ordinary obesity" differ from mutant obese mice and mutant obese humans in the critically important respects that they have high concentrations of leptin in blood, large deposits of fat, continue to seek food, and do not have obviously reduced metabolic rates but in most other respects are like their lean contemporaries. Specifically they have experienced normal growth and development. These facts have led to a postulation of "leptin resistance" or "leptin insensitivity". At least one mechanism of leptin resistance seems to be an impairment of movement of leptin from blood to the sites in the brain at which it has its characteristic effect [208].

Despite these discouraging facts the Amgen pharmaceutical company paid 25 million dollars for rights to leptin. Leptin resistance may be an explanation for the mixed results obtained in a clinical trial of injections of leptin in obese people. Sponsored by Amgen Inc. and the National Institutes of Health, Heymsfield and collaborators [209] gave daily injections of placebo and escalating doses of recombinant leptin to lean and obese people of both genders. Obese people were prescribed a diet calculated to provide a small Calorie deficit and slow weight loss. Lean people were treated for 4 weeks and obese people for 24 weeks. Both lean people and obese people lost some weight at 4 weeks on the largest dose of leptin. At 24 weeks some of the obese people receiving the largest doses lost quite significant amounts of weight, mostly fat, as estimated by dual energy X-ray absorptiometry. However there was large variation among individuals, ranging from small gains in weight to large losses. In the large dose cohort, while receiving injections, blood concentrations were manyfold higher than concentrations in the untreated state, even in obese people. There was no relationship between weight loss and base line concentrations of leptin in blood. The authors concluded that their study showed that administration of exogenous leptin appears to enhance weight loss in some obese subjects with elevated endogenous blood leptin concentrations but not all. Leptin resistance seems not absolute, at least in some obese persons.

Perhaps eventually a role for leptin will be found in the treatment of a group of people which may be larger than we now can know. A recent study reports the finding of thirteen persons in three families who had low but not absent leptin in blood, genetically mediated. Definite but not extreme obesity was present [210]. They differ from the people described above, reported by the same investigators, who have total leptin deficiency, by having only partial leptin deficiency and by seeming less obese. Perhaps leptin administration could be beneficial for such people.

Another group of people who might benefit from administration of leptin are those formerly obese people who by Calorie-restricted diets have been able to reduce to normal weight but have difficulty maintaining their reduced weight. Women who lost weight by dieting or bariatric surgery have been reported to have lower blood concentrations of leptin than an age and weight matched group and excised fat tissue from the postobese women secreted less leptin in vitro than the never obese group [211].

A second study of 12 weeks duration by Hukshorn and collaborators [212] included obese subjects given weekly subcutaneous injections of leptin chemically modified to make it absorbed into the blood slowly. Compared with a placebo-injected group, a hormone-injected group showed small elevations of blood leptin but no change in body weight or an array of metabolic characteristics. In neither the 24 week Heymsfield study nor the 12 week Hukshorn study were adverse effects other than local skin reactions at the injections sites observed.

Leptin appears not to be the antiobesity hormone. In addition to the apparent incongruity of persisting high concentrations of leptin in blood in the persisting presence of sometimes massive obesity, and ongoing large caloric intake, there is the fact leptin does not show an increased blood concentration during or immediately following meals [213]. Consequently, despite the history of the research leading to its discovery, it does not seem in any simple way to be a "satiety factor".

While leptin has been disappointing as an antiobesity hormone in humans it has an impressive relation to starvation. Blood concentrations fall perceptibly during less than one day of fasting and before clearly measurable weight loss occurs [214]. Plainly, factors in addition to fat mass influence the blood concentration of leptin. During sustained Calorie restriction resulting in weight loss and eventual stabilization of weight and energy balance blood leptin concentration is lower, and lower per unit of fat mass, at least in women, than at their usual weight [215] . Experiments in rodents and humans [216] suggest that lowered blood leptin resulting from fasting or sustained Calorie restriction relieves a tonic inhibition of food-seeking by normal or elevated blood leptin. According to this idea there is disinhibition of brain centers mediating food-seeking, via several neurohormones mentioned above. If food is available, fat mass and leptin rise to levels present before Calorie restriction began.

The concept of a system in which leptin, or any mechanism, provides little opposition to accumulation of fat but is effective in countering starvation accords well with current ideas about the evolution of man and other mammals. About 1.5 million years ago there lived in Africa a tool-using anthropoid, Homo erectus, presumed to be a hunter-gatherer, believed by many anthropologists to have evolved into our own species, Homo sapiens, perhaps about 150,000 years ago [217]. For most of the existence of our species our progenitors were hunter-gatherers until they invented agriculture, farming, and fixed residences about 10,000 years ago in North Africa. For the first time in the history of man food was constantly and probably more abundantly available. In the context of evolution 10,000 years is an almost insignificant interval. We, present day Homo sapiens, have the genome of hunter-gatherers evolved, by enhancement of reproductive success, in a world in which the food supply was unreliable and usually limited. Our ancestors had little need for a physiological mechanism which prevented accumulation of fat. Indeed, our survival, and reproduction were enhanced by the ability to store fat and energy in a milieu in which the food supply was probably frequently interrupted by drought, floods, pests, glaciations, fire and other natural causes.

Looking about yourself while strolling down the streets of the United State or, increasingly, Europe should convince you that some of us have genomes better adapted to a hunter-gatherer existence than others. People who tend to accumulate large amounts of body fat when food is constantly and abundantly available have been said to have a "thrifty genotype" and are assumed better to endure a hunting-gathering life than their constitutionally lean contemporaries in an environment in which the supply of food was limited and unreliable. Evolutionary aspects of obesity and related topics has been insightfully reviewed by Lev-Ran [218;219].

There has been much interest in the idea that thriftiness sometimes somehow results from programming by fetal under nutrition rather than genes in developing countries [88].

Despite initial disappointment there is interest in the possibility that leptin might in some way be used to help people to shed unwanted and unhealthy fat deposits. There are at least two serious negative features. The first is that presently available forms of the hormone must be injected to be effective. This may not be a decisive disincentive. Many obese people are highly motivated. A more serious problem is the possibility of serious adverse effects with prolonged administration. Leptin has a significant role in many physiological processes not discussed here. Included are reproductive development, maturation, and function, bone metabolism, and function of the autonomic nervous system.

The above paragraphs and figure present a view of leptin's physiology and of a group of rare genetic aberrations of leptin gene and leptin receptor gene with respect to obesity. The rapid advances which have occurred following the initial discoveries about leptin have revealed a system, complex and redundant, capable of exquisite sensitivity in the regulation of body adiposity. In the passages above we have considered only the quantity of leptin secreted and the integrity of the receptor which it activates. There must happen a multiplicity of events following activation of the receptor to reach the result of finely regulated feeding behavior, finely regulated metabolic activity, and finely regulated physical activity. There is now available some information concerning details of some of the downstream mechanisms which has led to the discovery of some new, but rare, genetic disorders. The knowledge amplifies our understanding of the mechanisms of regulation of fat depots and offers opportunities for pharmaceutical intervention.

The system is complex. I offer a pair of arrow diagrams which reveal, in a simplified way, what happens in the central nervous system, mediating peripheral metabolism, when leptin increases or decreases. Imagine that we have a steady state in which leptin secretion is intermediate, catabolism and anabolism are equal. Now suppose an episode of over-feeding. Adipose tissue is increased. Leptin secretion is increased, see Figure 2.

The increased leptin increases activation of the leptin receptor in the central nervous system. Neuropeptide Y production is diminished and ongoing activation of the neuropeptide Y receptor is diminished resulting in decreased anabolism by peripheral metabolic mechanisms. Alpha-melanocyte stimulating hormone production is increased, activating melanocortin 4 receptors, increasing peripheral catabolism. Agouti related peptide production is inhibited, relieving the disinhibition of the melanocyte 4 receptor, thus enhancing peripheral catabolism. Adipose tissue is restored to its former size.

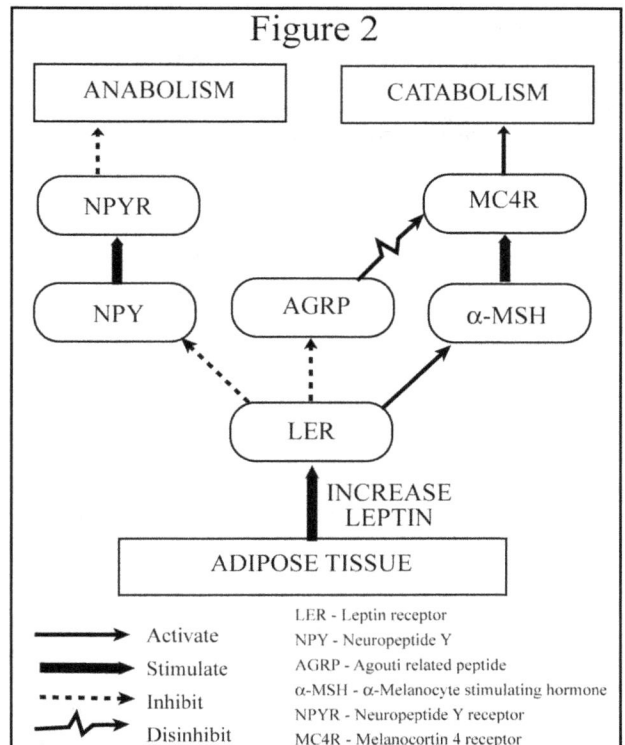

Figure 2

ANABOLISM   CATABOLISM

NPYR   MC4R

NPY   AGRP   α-MSH

LER

INCREASE LEPTIN

ADIPOSE TISSUE

→ Activate
⟹ Stimulate
----► Inhibit
⤳ Disinhibit

LER - Leptin receptor
NPY - Neuropeptide Y
AGRP - Agouti related peptide
α-MSH - α-Melanocyte stimulating hormone
NPYR - Neuropeptide Y receptor
MC4R - Melanocortin 4 receptor

Now suppose that the subject is fasted, see Figure 3 below.

Leptin production is diminished immediately, and before appreciable weight loss occurs. Neuropeptide Y secretion is increased peripheral mechanisms mediating anabolism manifest increased activity. At the same time agouti related peptide secretion is increased resulting in increased antagonism to the melanocortin 4 receptor. Alpha-melanocyte stimulating hormone production is diminished, further reducing activation of the melanocortin 4 receptor and inhibiting catabolism. Eventually adipose tissue and body fat are restored to their former size.

There are multiple sites in this system at which mutations causing loss of function could be expected to result in obesity. Genetic sources of obesity can be divided into three categories: 1) Polygenic obesity in which multiple genes contribute to accumulation of excess adipose tissue, common obesity, especially of the familial variety; 2) Monogenic obesity in which a mutation of a single gene results in loss of function creating a mechanism for obesity; and 3) Syndromic obesities in which obesity is only one of multiple clinically apparent disorders, assumed to be the consequence of often multiple mutations and chromosomal abnormalities.

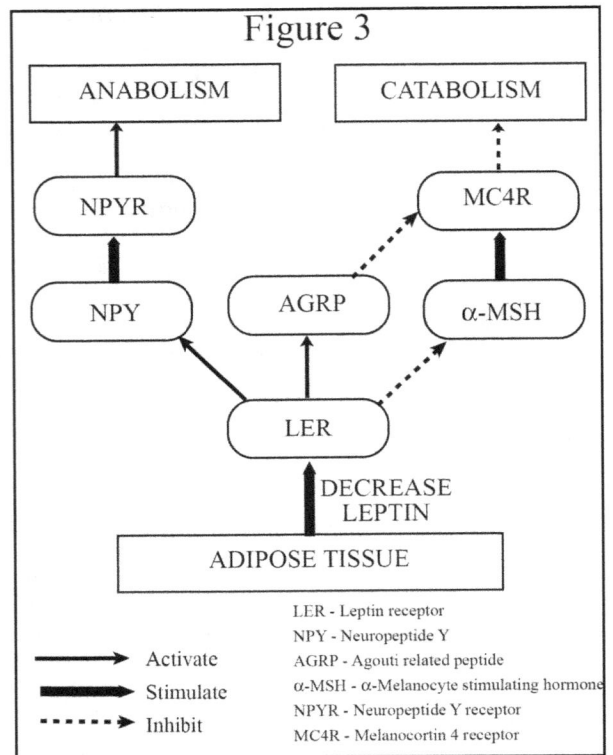

Figure 3

LER - Leptin receptor
NPY - Neuropeptide Y
AGRP - Agouti related peptide
α-MSH - α-Melanocyte stimulating hormone
NPYR - Neuropeptide Y receptor
MC4R - Melanocortin 4 receptor

→ Activate
⇒ Stimulate
----▶ Inhibit

The most common known monogenic variety of obesity is the consequence of one of several mutations of the gene for the melanocortin receptor 4 resulting in loss of function. From a clinical perspective, affected persons tend to be massively obese, always hungry, and taller than average, but otherwise grossly normal. There is often a history of early onset and frequently a family history of similar disorder. There have been several surveys of populations of obese persons assessing this gene [220-225]. Prevalence probably does not exceed 6% in the population most likely to have a mutation, persons with extreme obesity of early onset [226]. This computes to a small fraction of 1% in the general population [222]. Consequently melanocortin 4 receptor mutations cannot be considered an important problem from a public health perspective. However they are devastating for the affected individual. Study of monogenic mutations is justified by the understanding of the physiology of obesity which results.

The variability of the clinical picture, the preservation of reproductive function, and the detection of a variety of mutations of this gene have suggested that the MC4R gene has characteristics which would allow it, in concert with other genes, to play a central role in the production of the "thrifty" habitus [227]. The significance of some mutations of the MC4R gene is unclear. Tao and Segaloff have reported that *in vitro* testing of a variety of mutations has demonstrated the presence of loss-of-function variants in people who are not obese. This might be explained by the redundancy of the system regulating fat storage resulting in compensation for the loss of functional activity. They also found variants of the gene in obese people which did not result in loss of function suggesting that their obesity was not attributable to alteration of the MC4R gene [228]

The protein proopiomelanocortin (POMC) is synthesized in certain cells of the brain, encoded by a gene, in response to activation by leptin of the leptin receptor. It is undergoes sequential cleavage by a cascade of enzymes, each encoded by a gene, to several smaller peptides, including alpha-MSH. Mutation of the genes regulating the enzymes required for production of alpha-MSH could result in a faulty or insufficient product. The catabolic influence of the brain would then be diminished and unopposed influence of anabolic factors would cause obesity. One such mutation, encoding an enzyme named prohormone convertase 1, has been described in a person with extreme childhood-onset obesity and multiple endocrine and metabolic disorders [229]. Obesity can result from faulty processing of proopiomelanocortin by faulty enzymes and can also result from mutation of the gene encoding POMC which results in the production of a faulty substrate for those enzymes and insufficient or defective alpha-MSH. Two obese children with severe obesity and multiple endocrine and metabolic defects afflicted with mutation of the POMC gene have been detected [230].

A molecule similar to alpha-MSH, called beta-MSH, also occurs in humans. It has been believed that alpha-MSH is the functionally important molecule in people. However, five obese children have been described in whom beta-MSH was variant, suggesting that beta-MSH may have a role in weight-regulation in humans [231].

Of course mutations of genes for leptin and its receptor are monogenic obesities but are very rare.

The most convincing evidence for a genetic influence in "common" obesity, believed to be polygenic, comes from twin studies described above in the section labeled HEREDITY. There have been many studies suggesting that specific sites in the genome contribute to ordinary obesity. About 135 genes have been more or less credibly linked to obesity [232]. However, attempted replication of studies has often failed and there has been little understanding of the details of the mechanisms by which such genomic sites result in obesity. There are two major problems for researchers in this area. The first is that it seems likely that many genes are involved, each making a small contribution with different combinations in different people. The second is that while the genetic component is important, the production of obesity requires interaction with an environment which encourages consumption of large amounts of readily available food and exemption from much physical activity. It seems that the genes provide susceptibility and the environment brings about the obesity

A very large study published in 2009 reported that at least 8 genes are associated with increased BMI. None have a strong influence. Mechanisms by which they contribute to obesity are largely unknown though most are highly expressed in the central nervous system, suggesting that obesity is mediated mostly by the brain [233].

In 1999 there was described a previously unknown unusual and important hormonal protein, subsequently called ghrelin, secreted by the stomach of rats. A virtually identical substance is secreted by the stomachs of humans [234]. In humans, and rats, intravenously injected ghrelin promoted feeding under circumstances of ad lib food intake. Humans, (but not rats) said they had increased appetite while under the influence of the hormone [235]. In experiments with normal-weight subjects in which meals were scheduled at regular times, blood ghrelin concentration increased two fold before each meal and fell within one hour after eating. Secretion of ghrelin seems stimulated by a time-dependent signal, presumably neural, and inhibited by ingestion of food [236].

In obese persons the baseline, blood concentration of ghrelin is reduced and rises with diet-induced weight loss. The normal preprandial rise and postprandial decline in ghrelin levels are maintained before and after weight loss. The fasting concentration of ghrelin in blood negatively correlated with body fat mass estimated by dual X-ray absorptiometry. The relationship to body fat is present not only in obese persons but also in lean women [237]. As is leptin, ghrelin seems to be a monitor and index of body fat [238].

Although ghrelin is not a cause of obesity in a simple way it is important because it participates in the regulation of body fat depots by reason of its influence on appetite. Experiments in laboratory animals indicate that it exerts its effects by stimulating production of the neuroprotein Y/agouti-related protein complex in the central nervous system.

"GUT HORMONES", SATIETY FACTORS

Ghrelin is the first and only known orexigenic peptide originating outside the central nervous system. There are five known hormones which have an anorexigenic property, "satiety factors": peptide YY (3-

36) from the rectum and colon [239], pancreatic polypeptide coming mostly from the pancreas [240], oxyntomodulin from the small intestine, glucagon-like peptide-1 secreted by the small intestine, and cholecystokinin, also a product of the small intestine, collectively known as "gut hormones".

Peptide YY (3-36) seems to have a role in the regulation of food intake. This substance is secreted by the gastrointestinal tract in response to meals, in proportion to the caloric value of the meal. Intravenous injection in lean humans and in obese humans markedly diminishes appetite [241]. Fasting concentrations of the hormone in blood were low in obese persons, suggesting that Peptide YY may have a role in the production of obesity. Experiments in laboratory mice show that it acts through the proopiomelanocortin pathway [242].

Pancreatic polypeptide is a chemically similar substance, secreted by the pancreas and intestine in response to ingestion of food. When infused intravenously into nonobese humans it inhibits appetite and reduces *ad lib* food intake [243]. Reduced concentrations of the hormone in blood of obese persons have inconsistently been reported [244]. It is possible that pancreatic polypeptide participates in some way in the causation of some instances of obesity.
Oxyntomodulin, a hormone produced mostly by the small intestine, is secreted in response to meals [245]. Nonobese humans receiving intravenous infusions of oxyntomodulin manifested reduced food intake and suppression of ghrelin [246].

Glucagon-like peptide-1, secreted by the small intestine and pancreas in response to meals, responds less in obese persons than lean persons and the deficit is partially remedied by diet-mediated loss of 25% of body fat, assessed by dual X-ray absorptiometry [247]. Intravenous infusions of the hormone diminished *ad lib* food intake in both lean [248] and obese men [249].

Cholecystokinin is a hormone released by the small intestine in response to the presence of fats and amino acids (derivatives of dietary proteins) in the lumen of the duodenum, the upper part of the small intestine [250]. Intravenous infusions of the hormone inhibit food intake and hunger in both lean and obese subjects [251]. The effect is mediated, at least in part, by slowing of gastric emptying resulting in gastric fullness [252]. The state of the stomach is signaled to the brain by nerves innervating the abdominal viscera. Cholecystokinin seems to be involved also in a wide variety of behavioral phenomena, panic, anxiety, addiction and eating disorders [253]. (see **Eating Disorders** in **APPENDIX 2**)

Insulin, a hormone secreted by the intraabdominal pancreas, is thought to have a role in regulation of body fat which has not been satisfactorily delineated. More than 20 years ago it was shown by injections of insulin into various parts of the brains of rats and mice that the activity of insulin on structures of the central nervous system is anorexigenic resulting in weight loss although its peripheral extraneural action on fat cells is to stimulate fat synthesis and storage and consequently to promote weight gain [254-256]. Mice genetically engineered to be neuron-specifically unresponsive to insulin become obese [255]. There seems to be no definite consensus about the physiological role of insulin in regulation of body fat in humans. The action on the central nervous system has potential practical importance because conceivably a drug could be developed which mimics the action of insulin on the brain but has no extraneural effect on fat cells, an appetite suppressant [257]. (see **Insulin** in **APPENDIX 2**)

The "gut hormones" described above are released into the blood and thereby reach the brain and peripheral nerves where they exert their characteristic actions. They are released in response to mechanical stimuli, distention, presence of substances in the lumen of the gastrointestinal tract, and the presence of specific nutrients in the gastrointestinal tract.

In addition to the above described chemical messengers to the brain concerning events in the gastrointestinal tract, the signaling system of sensory nerves innervating the stomach and intestines carries nerve impulses to the brain. The nerves are stimulated by distention of the organs and by the presence of specific nutrients in the lumens of the organs and promote termination of feeding [258]. There is a large and difficult literature concerning the satiating effects of the different food substrates, protein, carbohydrate and fat, an obviously important topic. The topic is difficult because some of the many variables which must be considered are the nutritional state of the subject, the psychosocial matrix in which food ingestion occurs, the palatability and texture of the food and the caloric density of the food. Perhaps most students of this subject would agree that, all things being equal, protein has an efficient and effective satiating effect (satiation per Calorie ingested), carbohydrate some what less but significant, and fat very little. This rank-ordering is supported by a finding of a similar rank-ordering for suppression of blood ghrelin by ingested nutrients [259].

The lesser satiating effect of fat is appropriate in an evolutionary sense. If our hunter-gatherer ancestors were subject to episodes of severely reduced availability of food, liberal ingestion of fat, when available, would have survival value. This is because protein is not stored in our bodies; carbohydrate is stored in only very small amounts as liver glycogen but fat can be stored in calorically very large amounts and is readily available to supply needs
for energy.

The redundancy of this system presents an important challenge to researchers attempting to develop drugs for the treatment of obesity. Enhancement or inhibition of any component of the system may result in compensating inhibition or enhancement of some other component, preventing the expected consequences of change in any one component.
Much work remains to be done to achieve a comprehensive view of the regulation of body fat but there has been much progress. Intuitively, it seems that obtaining a thorough understanding of the system would be helpful or even indispensable for developing drugs or other devices for the prevention or management of obesity. A systems analytic way of thinking about the regulation of body fat postulates that body fat is regulated and relatively constant over long intervals despite significant day-to-day alterations of energy intake and energy expenditure, that the regulatory system includes long term components, leptin and possibly insulin, and that the system includes short term components, ghrelin and satiety factors [260]. Long term components stabilize body fat over intervals of months and years. Short term components regulate meal-to-meal energy economy. Perhaps some day there will be a mathematical model of obesity which will make possible individualized, quantitative assessment of causative mechanisms in obese people, guiding remediation in an individualized way.

SYNDROMIC OBESITIES

Certain rare disorders of development, genomically mediated, which include, among many signs, symptoms, clinical findings, and characteristic features, obesity are called syndromic obesities. Each syndrome is named for the persons who first published a description of it.

The most common appears to be the Prader-Willi syndrome. The incidence has been variably estimated at 1 in 10,000 live births to 1 in 22,000. Intensive study of such rare people is warranted by the belief that an understanding of the mechanisms governing their development will be helpful in approaching people with more common disorders. Children born with the Prader-Willi syndrome are short, massively obese with an insatiable appetite, mentally deficient, and hypogonadal, displaying retarded or absent development of sexual organs and function. Abnormalities of growth and sexual function are attributable to maldevelopment of the hypothalamus which fails to mediate secretion of growth hormone and the hormones necessary for normal development of sexual organs and function. Localization of at least part of the disturbed mechanism to the hypothalamus suggests the hypothesis that obesity and food-seeking might be the result of altered function of neuropeptide Y, agouti-related protein, alpha melanocyte stimulating hormone, leptin, ghrelin or some combination thereof. Leptin concentrations in blood and generation of leptin receptor in Prader-Willi women seem similar to those of similarly obese "normal" women of similar age [261]. Blood ghrelin concentrations in children with Prader-Willi syndrome are several fold higher than those in "normal" children matched for age, gender, and body mass index [262]. The mechanism for the increased ghrelin concentrations is unknown. However, it seems that increased ghrelin in blood is at least partially the cause of excessive appetite and adiposity in the Prader-Willi syndrome. Additionally, rise in blood concentrations of the anorexigen pancreatic polypeptide in response to feeding is reduced [263]. Intravenous infusion of pancreatic polypeptide reduced food intake of children with the Prader-Willi syndrome [264].

The genes responsible for the syndrome are not known. The Prader-Willi syndrome is the result, usually, of defective expression of genes of the chromosome 15 contributed by the male parent. The gene for ghrelin is on chromosome 3. The gender distribution of the syndrome is equal [265].

The Angelman syndrome, small head, prominent nose and mouth, ataxia and severe obesity, is the consequence, usually, of defective expression of genes of the chromosome 15 contributed by the female parent [266].

The rare Bardet-Beidl syndrome consists of severe obesity, retinitis pigmentosa (a progressive degenerative disorder of the retina), polydactyly (supernumerary fingers and toes), mental deficiency, deformed urinary tract and hypogenitalism. Family pedigrees manifest a clear pattern of inheritance with a prevalence ranging from 1 in 160,000 in Switzerland through 1 in 16,000 in Newfoundland to 1 in 13,500 in Kuwaiti Bedouins[267]. Prevalence is enhanced in populations in which consanguinity is enhanced by geographical or cultural isolation. The syndrome is clinically heterogeneous indicating complex genetic backgrounds. The latter characteristic, reminiscent of "ordinary obesity", has inspired the interest of the research community [268]. There are 8 recognized subtypes, one of which has been persuasively associated with a particular gene [269].

Some other, less thoroughly studied, heritable syndromes including obesity are the Alstrom syndrome (obesity, retinal degeneration, nerve deafness, diabetes mellitus, type II, and cardiac degeneration), the Cohen syndrome (obesity, small head and mental deficiency), and the Carpenter syndrome (obesity, mental deficiency, male hypogenitalism, cephalic deformity and polydactyly).

Narcolepsy is a rare syndrome characterized by sleep disorder, episodic generalized paralysis without loss of consciousness and a tendency to moderate obesity. The prevalence has been estimated to be 1 in 2,000 in Europe and the United States [270]. Most of current belief about it has come from elegant experiments in dogs, rats, and mice. In dogs narcolepsy is the result of mutation of a gene. In rats and mice it is produced by genetic modification in the laboratory and in humans it is the result of an unexplained progressive death of certain cells in the brain, neurons which signal other neurons by secretion of a peptide called orexin A. In all species narcolepsy is the consequence of deficiency of orexin A. Additional characteristics of narcolepsy are obesity despite diminished spontaneous food intake. Metabolic rate and physical activity are diminished [271]. All manifestations are reversed by administration of orexin A. Orexin fibers project to areas of the brain in which the neurohormones NPY, AGRP, and alpha-MSH are functioning and to areas of the brain which mediate arousal, vigilance, attentiveness (see Figure 2).

Obviously not much of our rising prevalence of obesity can be attributed to frank orexin deficiency. However, the findings in narcolepsy bring to mind the observations concerning reduced "spontaneous physical activity" [166] and reduced "nonexercise activity thermogenesis" [164] as risk factors for obesity. Perhaps in some complex way orexin neurons play a role in some forms of obesity not now recognized. Whether that is true or not think of this arresting possibility: Suppose there were available a procedure or drug which enhanced or mimicked the action of orexin A. Perhaps obese persons could enjoy more food, more physical activity and less adiposity.

VISCERAL OBESITY

In 1932 the celebrated neurosurgeon Harvey Cushing described a disorder which not surprisingly came to be called Cushing's syndrome. Manifestations include elevated blood pressure, a tendency to diabetes mellitus type II, and a peculiar distribution of adipose tissue in which the extremities are thin, the face is rounded ("moon face"), the shoulders and upper back are padded with fat ("buffalo hump"), and there is upper abdominal obesity ("pot belly") subsequently known as android obesity or visceral obesity. In the decade following Cushing's description of this syndrome much was learned about the chemistry, physiology, biological activities and metabolism of the hormones of the adrenal cortex. It was soon established that the disorder is attributable to excessive secretion by the adrenal cortex of a substance now called cortisol, a major inactive metabolite of which is called cortisone.

In 1947 a publication by the French clinician Vague [272] made the point that, indeed, there is a difference between men and women. Obese women tend to accumulate fat around thighs, hips, lower abdomen and buttocks. Obese men tend to have a protuberant upper abdomen. By 1957 that same observant clinician [273] was promoting recognition of the now well established association of upper body obesity with diabetes mellitus type II and vascular disease.

The similarities between patients with Cushing's syndrome , especially in milder instances, and men, commonly seen in every clinician's office, with protuberant abdomens, (intraabdominal obesity), diabetes mellitus type II, and coronary heart disease, immediately stimulated the interest of clinical investigators. As practical, accurate, specific chemical assays for cortisol and its metabolites became available, a large literature accumulated. It described experiments designed to elucidate the role of cortisol in obesity. Data were sometimes difficult to interpret and were sometimes inconsistent. However, during an interval of years there developed consensus about two matters. Firstly, concentrations of cortisol in blood of obese people do not consistently differ from those in comparable lean persons and are consistently lower than those in people with Cushing's syndrome. Secondly, measurements of cortisol and its metabolites in urine indicate that obese persons secrete more cortisol than lean persons, in proportion to the extent to which they are overweight. The latter finding can plausibly be attributed to the known larger actively metabolizing fat-free mass of obese persons. These conclusions do not support a belief that cortisol plays a role in the development of obesity. However, in 1997 there appeared a paper which offered new insights. The paper, by Bujalska, Kumar, and Stewart, [274] was entitled "Does central obesity reflect 'Cushing's disease of the omentum'?" (The omentum is a large membranous supporting structure within the abdomen which even in lean persons contains significant amounts of fat and in obese persons contains very large amounts of fat.)

Biologically active cortisol, secreted by the adrenal cortex, is converted to biologically inactive cortisone by an enzyme called 11β-hydroxysteroid dehydrogenase type 2. The enzyme is widely distributed in tissues. It is found in kidney, pancreas, and intestine. Active cortisol is regenerated from cortisone by an enzyme called 11β-hydroxysteroid dehydrogenase type 1 which is found in liver, lung, spleen, brain, and adipose tissue. The special contribution of Bujalska and colleagues was the demonstration that, in tissue biopsies, 11β-hydroxysteroid dehydrogenase type 1 activity tends to be relatively greater in omental fat than subcutaneous fat. The significance of this finding is that the exposure of adipocytes in omental fat to cortisol can exceed that of adipocytes in subcutaneous tissue. Cortisol promotes differentiation of preadipocytes to adipocytes and the deposition of fat in adipocytes [275]. These facts provide a basis for a hypothetical description of a continuum of visceral obesity to generalized or to gynecoid obesity, namely a continuum of relative preponderance of 11β-hydroxysteroid dehydrogenase type 1 activity in intraabdominal fat over that in subcutaneous fat.

Strong support for the above idea has come from experiments with inbred genetically engineered mice. The animals were genetically modified to express increased activity of 11β-hydroxysteroid dehydrogenase activity type 1 exclusively in adipose tissue [276] . They ate more than comparable mice, gained more weight and had a larger percentage of fat in their abdomens than comparable mice. They were diabetic and had increased metabolic risk factors for vascular disease, a topic to be discussed in the next chapter. In summary, the modified mice closely resembled the commonly seen people who have visceral obesity, diabetes mellitus type II and vascular disease.

These findings are important, exciting, because although intraabdominal adipose tissue is small in quantity it is large in consequence. In men visceral fat is about 20% of total body fat and in women about 6% [277]. Nevertheless visceral obesity is a critically important risk factor for morbidity and mortality from diabetes mellitus type II, hypertension, heart attacks, strokes and other vascular catastrophes. Further, we now have a demonstration that, contrary to previous assumptions, all fat cells are not the same. Adipose tissue is not merely a depository for fat but is a varied, complex system which interacts with other tissues and organs in ways additional to those resulting from its deposition and release of fat and its metabolites and does so in a region-specific way. Last but not least is the idea that this understanding may lead to measures to prevent illness.

Immediately a question comes to mind: What are the risk factors for development of increased visceral adipose tissue? Answers to this question are not completely satisfying because the most trusted means of indexing visceral adipose tissue are computer assisted tomography (CAT scans) and magnetic resonance imaging (MRI). Reservations concerning these methods will be discussed in succeeding chapters but it is sufficient to write at this point that the technologies require large, expensive machines and trained, skilled personnel and are thus unsuitable for large epidemiological surveys similar to studies, for example, employing the body mass index. This is important because the deposition of visceral fat, i.e. the mechanism productive of abdominal adiposity, is a multifactorial phenomenon. The consequence is that large volumes of quality data are required for the optimal elucidation of complex interrelationships, which may be for any given individual, unique. However, despite the difficulties, there seem to be some observable trends. Important known influences to be considered are gender, the level of generalized adiposity, age, and genes.

At any given level of total body adiposity men have a larger amount of intraabdominal adipose tissue than women and the fraction of total adiposity which is intraabdominal is greater in men than in women [278]. Men tend to be "apple-shaped" and women tend to be "pear-shaped". This is a statistical relation. There are many men who are pear-shaped, i.e. have predominantly subcutaneous adipose deposits of the lower abdomen, buttocks and thighs. There are many women who are apple-shaped, i.e. have predominantly upper intraabdominal adipose deposits. People who have large deposits of total body fat have larger deposits of intraabdominal fatty tissue but also have larger deposits of subcutaneous fat and are not necessarily apple-shaped.

The sexual dimorphism for visceral adipose tissue suggests a role for sex hormones. There appears to be one but it is not what one might intuitively expect and it is not well understood. In men the principal source of male hormones, called androgens, is the testes. The adrenal cortex contributes small amounts of androgen. In men, both the testes and the adrenal cortex are the source of small amounts of female hormones, called estrogens. In women the principal source of estrogens is the ovaries, which also produce small amounts of androgen. Also in women, the adrenal cortex is the source of small amounts of androgen and estrogen. Testicular production of androgen declines in men as they age. In women, menopause signals the rather abrupt cessation of ovarian estrogen production.

When the potent androgen, testosterone, is administered to men, visceral adipose tissue is reduced [279]. Men with larger amounts of intraabdominal adipose tissue tend to have lower concentrations of testosterone in blood although the values may be within the range considered to be normal [280]. In experiments in which radio-isotope labeled fat was given orally to men undergoing abdominal surgery and assimilation of lipid radioactivity into visceral fat was measured in biopsies, it was shown that administration of testosterone inhibited incorporation of orally administered fat into intraabdominal fat [281]. When visceral adipose tissue is increased metabolic features associated with cardiovascular disease are more prevalent [282]. As men age and testicular secretion of androgen decreases, intraabdominal adipose tissue increases. It may be that the loss of a protective effect of testicular androgen accounts for the increasing abdominal adiposity observed in men as they age.

What is the effect of androgen on visceral adipose tissue in women? An investigator could not ethically administer a substantially effective amount of androgen to normal women because the effect of androgen on hair is to a significant extent irreversible. What normal woman wants a beard and bald scalp? To avoid this dilemma Elbers and associates [283] made observations in an unusual group of women, female-to-male transsexuals. These often very unhappy people seem by every medical criterion to be normal women but have a passionate, determined desire to assume in every possible way a male identity. They eagerly undergo surgery to remove breasts and reconstruct genitalia. Androgen is administered in effective quantity to convert skin and hair and other organs to a male pattern. When this is done they manifest an increase in visceral adiposity.

An apparently rare experiment of nature confirms that the abdominal consequence of administering androgens to female-to-male transsexuals is not a mere clinical artifact but is representative of physiological reality. A complex, genetically mediated disorder of hormone metabolism, called cortisone reductase deficiency, has the consequence of increased secretion of androgens by the adrenal glands. When this occurs in women it is accompanied by abdominal obesity [284]. .Postmenopausal women have larger amounts of visceral adipose tissue than premenopausal women [285] and larger amounts of visceral adipose tissue are correlated with larger concentrations of androgens in blood [286] Data from Japan suggest that administration of usual hormone replacement therapy (oral conjugated equine estrogen and medroxy progesterone acetate) to postmenopausal women inhibits the expected increase in visceral fatty tissue, measured by computer assisted tomography, only in women with an initial android distribution of fat,[287]. It may not, in so doing, diminish risk of coronary heart disease [288]. These hormones given to a large group of American postmenopausal women without respect to the amount of body fat or its distribution resulted in a small increase in coronary artery disease by comparison with an appropriate control group of women. It is not known what might occur in women with large amounts of visceral adipose tissue or predisposed to the development of visceral adiposity.

The adrenal cortex and the ovaries secrete a substance named androstenedione which can be converted by adipose tissue either to the prototypical male hormone, testosterone, or to female hormones, estrogens. Recent evidence indicates that in women the capacity of the mechanisms of intraabdominal fatty tissue locally to produce testosterone from androstenedione exceeds the capacity to produce estrogen and does so increasingly as intraabdominal adipose tissue increases. It appears that in women the presence of intraabdominal fat enhances the deposition of intraabdominal fat.

In women, moderate alcohol ingestion is associated with larger deposits of visceral adipose tissue and increased concentration in blood of testosterone [289]

The superficial facts are, in summary, in genetic males, androgen hormones protect against growth of intraabdominal adipose tissue and, in genetic females, androgen hormones promote growth of intraabdominal adipose tissue. In genetic females estrogen protects against deposition of intraabdominal fat.

Aging results in an increase in body weight, in total body fat, especially visceral adipose tissue, and a decrease in fat-free mass. As described above, the increase in visceral adiposity is mediated, at least in part, by age-associated changes in sex hormones. However, aging is a risk factor for increased central adiposity independent of menopause. Increasing visceral adipose tissue begins in middle-aged women before the onset of menopause [290]. Increased total fat seems attributable to several factors. Surely a part of the explanation is reduced physical activity perhaps related to diminished muscle mass [46;291]. An age-correlated decline in circulating leptin, in both genders, despite an age-correlated rise in total body fat may contribute to increased body weight and increased total fat [292] in the same way that a fasting-mediated decline in blood leptin enhances food-seeking behavior and anabolic mechanisms (see Figure 3).

A prospective 5 year study of Americans aged 70 to 79 showed that symptoms of depression, indexed by standardized testing, predicts development of visceral obesity, measured by computerized tomography, independent of change in Body Mass Index [293]. It is plausible to speculate that this finding reflects a change in cortisol secretion or metabolism. See cortisol above.

Additional factors contributing to weight gain and increased adiposity with aging appear to be reduced mobilization of fat stores in response to exercise and sympathetic hormones [294], reduced resting metabolic rate partially attributable to reduced fat-free mass[295], reduced diet-induced thermogenesis attributable to reduced sensitivity to stimulation by sympathetic hormones [296;297], and reduced increase of fat metabolism mediated by exercise and sympathetic stimulation [298;299].

It is commonly observed that women tend to be more adipose than men. In fact, measurements by densitometry and other means uniformly show women have a larger proportion of body weight as fat than men and, on average, carry a larger absolute fat mass than men. Of course, they must have a smaller fat-free mass than men since, on average, they weigh less. Consequently, female gender can be thought to be a risk factor for obesity, no matter how defined. These facts are consistent with the findings that women, while tending to live a physically less active life, have a lower daily energy expenditure, statistically corrected for age, fat mass, and fat-free mass [300].

At age 6 years children born small for gestational age tend to be viscerally obese in both genders in comparison with same-weight contemporaries. The mechanism for this is unknown and it is not known whether the visceral adiposity persists into adulthood [301].

SUMMARY AND CONCLUSIONS

A very large number of people, perhaps most people, have a genetically mediated, heritable, susceptibility to the development of obesity in an environment of easily accessible abundant food and absence of requirements for physical activity. A small number of people have a genetically mediated, heritable, resistance to the development of obesity. The molecular mechanisms underlying both susceptibility and resistance are poorly understood but appear to be multiple, redundant, and varied. The pattern of mechanisms may vary from person to person as do other attributes. The intensity of both susceptibility and resistance is highly varied in the population.

Research in this field is difficult because of the complexity of the biochemical, and physiological, systems and the practical obstacles to maintaining consistent defined experimental conditions in humans for a sufficiently long time to arrive at firm conclusions. Laboratory animal models have been very helpful in indicating the presence of relevant mechanisms.

CHAPTER FOUR: MEDICAL HAZARDS OF OBESITY

The medical hazards of obesity are appalling but are not the only hazards of obesity. Many people feel keenly the psychosocial, economic and other consequences. In the United States and Europe obese people experience discrimination in employment, education, health care [302] and other important aspects of life [303]. While bias is most obviously directed against women, men are not immune [304]. Such psychosocial handicaps begin early in life. Obese children are sometimes treated with contempt and hostility by their lean contemporaries [305].

A measure of the way in which obesity intrudes into every facet of the lives of all of us, obese or lean, can be found in the estimate that annual obesity-related medical expenditures in the United States have been about $75 billion, in 2003 dollars, about one half financed by Federal government programs, Medicaid and Medicare [306]. Obesity-related annual hospital costs for children aged 6 to 17 years have been estimated to have increased more than threefold, comparing the interval 1979-1981 with the interval 1997-1999 [307]. "Increases in the proportion of (spending) and (of) spending on obese people relative to people of normal weight account for 27 percent of the rise in inflation-adjusted per capita spending between 1987 and 2001..."[15].

An elevated body mass index in young adulthood and middle age is associated with greatly increased medical expenditures in the same people when they are aged 65 years or older [308]. Health care costs of obese adults are greater than those of nonobese adults, mostly as a consequence of costs of prescription drugs [309]

In the pages to follow while focusing on the medical hazards we should not forget that we are examining only part of the harmful features of obesity. There are several serious defects in the voluminous literature relating obesity to health. One is almost exclusive reliance on the body mass index (weight in kilograms divided by height in meters squared, BMI) as an index of body fat. Characteristics of the BMI have been discussed in the chapter with the heading "How is Obesity Measured?". It is not an index of body fat but an index of body weight. It is mathematically biased and its relationship to body fat is influenced by age, gender, and ethnicity/race [55;310;311]. It provides no information about the regional distribution of body fat. Nevertheless it is the most commonly employed index of body fat in epidemiological studies and for some surveys probably offers the only practical datum. It is readily available, accurate, and inexpensive. There have been efforts to develop a substitute but the body mass index has continued to be the most frequently used tool [312;313].

In 1998 the National Heart, Lung and Blood Institute in a clinical guideline promulgated a definition of obesity as a BMI of 30 or greater and defined overweight as a BMI of 25 or greater [314] in adults. The choice of BMI 25 as threshold for overweight and BMI 30 as threshold for obese was based on studies indicating that "epidemiological data...show increases in mortality with BMIs above 25 kg/m^2. The increase in mortality, however tends to be modest until a BMI of >30 kg/m^2 is reached" [314]. The epidemiological data mentioned were derived mostly from surveys of American adults of various age, gender, and ethnic/racial characteristics and therefore may not have equally valid application to other populations [315-317]. These definitions have a degree of arbitrariness in that the risk of morbidity and mortality relative to body fat is a continuum rather than a sharply inflected phenomenon. A similar classification has been adopted by the World Health Organization [318].

A second serious defect is that most studies are cross-sectional, survey, case control or correlational studies. Obese persons and lean persons from a population of interest are examined for a morbidity of interest. If the pathology is more prevalent in the obese group it may be said that obesity and the morbidity are correlated. However, without additional information, it cannot be confidently determined whether the obesity is the cause of the morbidity, or the morbidity is the cause of obesity, or obesity and the morbidity are not causally related but are the consequence of some other factor or factors. A superior but more difficult study is the prospective or cohort study in which a representative sample of the population of interest is chosen and examined before obesity or the morbidity has developed and examined at later times when the morbidity and/or obesity have developed.

An example of the problem is found in the coprevalence of obesity and a major form of arthritis, osteoarthritis. Does this mean that arthritis, limiting physical activity, is a risk factor for obesity, or does it mean that obesity, over-loading joints, is a risk factor for osteoarthritis, or both or neither?

MORTALITY

A looming hazard of excess body fat is loss of life, a recognized, easily determined phenomenon. Although it has been stated for 2500 years that obesity is associated with excess mortality, published studies systematically documenting the phenomenon did not appear until the third decade of the twentieth century. Not surprisingly and appropriately they emanated from the life insurance industry. The first detailed survey, published in 1930, of large numbers of persons taking account of age, cause of death and body weight relative to average body weight of the population of men surveyed was that by Dublin of the Metropolitan Life Insurance Company [319]. Some important factors not considered were a more specific index of body fat, gender, socioeconomic measures, ethnicity/race, and smoking. Nevertheless the author was able to present some critical and durable conclusions: too light may be bad, too heavy is definitely bad, as a risk factor for cardiovascular disease.

In the 70 years since Dublin's pioneering survey there have been many studies of the relationship of body fat to all-cause mortality. There are many confounding, complicating variables. Among them are: smoking, degree of adiposity, gender, age, race/ethnicity, and cardiovascular fitness.

There has been little doubt that frank obesity is associated with risk for premature death. Peeters found that forty year old obese female nonsmokers lost 7.1 years of life expectancy and forty year old obese male nonsmokers lost 5.8 years of life expectancy by comparison with normal weight nonsmokers [320]. Assessing the presumed additive effect of smoking has been difficult because smoking tends to reduce weight but also is a risk factor for lethal disease [320-325].

At any BMI and any age up to 75 years men tend to experience somewhat greater all-cause mortality than do women [326]. For adults of both genders the all-cause relative risk of death attributable to increasing BMI is attenuated with advancing age (relative to the same-age people who have the BMI of lowest risk) and nearly disappears after age 75 years except in those with BMI greater than 32 [315;327]. In people aged 70 to 75 years the lowest risk for all-cause mortality occurs in the overweight by BMI category [328]. With respect to Federal guidelines it has been suggested that "Future guidelines should consider the evidence for specific age groups when establishing standards for healthy weight" [329].

A prospective study of Southwest American Indian children, aged 5 to 19, years, found that children in the highest quartile for BMI were significantly more likely to experience premature death, before age 55 years, than those in the lower quartile categories [330].

In a large Swedish study, among women developing breast cancer, cancer-specific mortality was not related to BMI except in women taking hormone replacement therapy. In those women those with BMI 30 or greater clearly experienced greater cancer-specific mortality than those with BMI less than 30 [331].

Statistically adjusted for age, BMI-correlated risk for all-cause mortality is less in African-Americans of both genders than in Caucasians [326]. There is, however, clear BMI-associated risk of diabetes mellitus type II and hypertension in African-Americans as in Caucasians, at least in women [332].

There have been few studies which directly addressed the issue of all-cause mortality with respect to adiposity and cardiovascular fitness. This is important for many people who have been unable to reduce body fat might wonder if attaining fitness would provide the same benefit with respect to mortality. In a large study of mostly middle-aged men, measuring body fat by densitometry and skin fold thickness, and cardiovascular fitness by a treadmill test, fitness reduced the *all-cause mortality* of men with the highest fat mass to that seen in fit men with the lowest fat mass. However, fitness failed to reduce *cardiovascular mortality* in men with high fat mass to the level observed in fit men with low fat mass [333]. This result has been confirmed [334]. In another large study of middle-aged men and women assessing fatness by BMI, and fitness by treadmill testing, the results showed that "both fitness and fatness are risk factors for mortality, and being fit does not completely reverse the increased risk associated with excess adiposity" [335]. A very large study of adults older than 60 years demonstrated that all cause mortality is associated with low level fitness (treadmill test) independently of adiposity (BMI, underwater weighing, skinfolds) A plausible conclusion from these data is that fitness provides benefits, may extend life at any level of fatness, but perhaps does not fully eliminate the deleterious effects of obesity. Even in older persons the benefits of fitness may justify a recommendation for exercise [336].

No one seriously doubts that persons with BMI equal to or greater than 30 (obese) have significant risk of premature mortality. However there has been question about the extent of risk for persons having BMI 25 to 29.9 (overweight). In 2005 a report by Flegal and associates [337] attracted much journalistic attention, some of it with a distinct tone of *Schadenfreude.* The report alleged that nearly all strictly excess fat-attributable deaths of adults in the United States in the year 2000 occurred in frankly obese persons, BMI equal to or greater than 30, and that the number is much smaller than any previous estimate, about 112,000 in the year 2000, far less than the 365,000 for the same year reported by Mokdad and associates [338]. (Published correction: JAMA 2005; 293:298.) Excess fat-attributable mortality declined with time in persons participating in surveys conducted 1971-1975, 1976-1980 and 1988-1994 and was virtually confined in every survey examined to persons with BMI 30 or larger. Of great interest to all concerned was the finding that being "overweight", defined by the Federal guideline, BMI 25 to 29.9, was *not* associated with excess obesity-attributable mortality in any of the surveys and, indeed, was associated with somewhat reduced mortality in comparison with "normal weight" (BMI 18.5 – 24.9) persons. Multiple earlier reports, including some of those cited above, have alleged significant increased excess mortality associated with BMI 25-25.9 [322;339]. Flegal and associates suggested that improvements in health care, especially for cardiovascular disease and the risk factors, high blood cholesterol, high blood pressure and smoking, may account, at least partially, for reduced risk of obesity-attributable mortality in persons with BMI 30 or greater. Gregg and associates studied the same populations described in Flegal and associates report [340]. They found a steady decrease with time in blood cholesterol, blood pressure and smoking. They also found a steady increase with time in use of medicines to lower blood cholesterol and blood pressure. The greatest changes were found in the heaviest people.

The report by Flegal and associates differed from most previous reports in significant ways. Advanced statistical procedures were used to account for the influence of the confounding factors age, gender, smoking, race, and alcohol use in an attempt to make the results more truly obesity-specific, *i.e.* to obtain a result attributable to obesity without the influence of the covariates gender, smoking, race, and alcohol use. The data bases employed were constructed to be representative of the whole United States population. The authors were not reluctant to point out the limitations of their study. Some of the coefficients used in their calculations were derived from decades-old data. Although they attempted to cope with the confounders, gender, smoking, race, age and alcohol, there are numerous other possible influences which were not addressed, *e.g.* diet, family history, physical exertion and coincidental disease..

There have been several previous less elaborate studies with results indicating similar conclusions [324;341] [325;342;343]. The Flegal report should have little impact on medical practice for the Federal guide lines promulgated in 1998 recommended treatment for weight loss for persons with BMI 25.0-29.9 only if 2 or more risk factors for cardiovascular disease, diabetes mellitus type II, smoking, high blood pressure, physical inactivity are present [314]. There is no apparent reason to change this. There is danger that persons in this weight category who are unaware of their risk factors may find false solace in incomplete popular media accounts of the Flegal report. The information in this report, if confirmed, could be seen as good news by the innumerable persons having a BMI of 30 or more who have been unable to lose weight for it seems that they can reduce the risk of death without weight loss by controlling blood pressure, blood cholesterol and other risk factors for cardiovascular disease and avoiding smoking and alcohol abuse. However, any comfort derived from this belief is considerably attenuated by evidence that even in persons overweight, BMI 25-29.9, and also in persons obese, BMI 30 or greater, there is substantially increased prevalence of diabetes mellitus type II, gallbladder disease, coronary heart disease, high blood cholesterol, high blood pressure, and osteoarthritis [344]. An additional important fact is that young people aged 20 to 22 years who are overweight, BMI 25-29.9, are significantly more likely to become obese, BMI 30 or greater, at age 35 to 37 years than are their contemporaries with BMI less than 25 [345].

Not surprisingly it seems likely that modern medicine has made it possible to live longer though chronically diseased. See the list of comorbidities below (also see **Comorbidities** in **APPENDIX 2**). Consistent with this point of view is the finding in a prospective study that overweight (BMI 25.0 – 29.9) in young adulthood and middle age is associated with increased Medicare costs in those persons when they are 65 years of age or older [308] . Additional support comes from a study showing that rising spending of private health insurance, inflation-adjusted, is to a significant extent attributable to treated disease prevalence, rather than increased cost per treated case, with disorders associated with obesity prominently represented [346].

Subsequent to the report by Flegal and collaborators there have appeared two high quality studies which seemed to show increased mortality in the BMI category 25–29.9, overweight, and confirming previous reports that low BMI and BMI 30 or greater are associated with excess mortality. In a large group of Americans aged 50-71 years of age in 1995-1996 excess mortality was reported in the group having BMI 25-29.9 at followup in the year 2000 [347]. In a large group of Koreans living in Korea, aged 30-95 years, excess mortality associated with BMI 25-29.9 was reported after 12 years of followup [348].

None of these studies is precisely comparable to any other. Differences include different populations with respect to race/ethnicity, gender, age, diet, coexisting morbidities, trajectory of BMI over time, smoking, alcohol consumption, the relation of BMI to adiposity and the regional distribution of fat. Consequently the presence of numerous conflicts of data and of interpretation in the literature of the epidemiology of obesity is not surprising. Regional distribution of fat seems especially important. There is evidence that for any given BMI mortality is closely related to waist circumference, a proxy for visceral adipose tissue [349]. A large multinational study demonstrated that waist circumference and waist-to-hip circumference ratio are more closely related to the risk of heart attack (myocardial infarction) than is BMI [350].

Although details of excess-fat-attributable mortality are difficult to establish they are important for developing public health policy. Additional research may refine knowledge of how obesity relates to mortality [351]. Although there is uncertainty concerning the extent of the risk of death associated with BMI 25-29.9 there is no doubt of increased risk of diabetes mellitus type II, hypertension and a host of morbidities. Persons with BMI in this range would be prudent to avoid additional weight gain.

MISCELLANEOUS COMORBIDITIES

A large array of morbidities has been attributed to obesity. In many instances the data supporting the attribution are not fully conclusive in that the studies have been correlational, cross sectional, in design. However in some instances the surveys are of cohort prospective design and the conclusions are firm. Below is a table providing selected information about selected comorbidities (see **APPENDIX 2**). The tabulated list of comorbidities is not comprehensive. Items were chosen on grounds of their importance to persons afflicted and the quality of evidence indicating the association.

In most instances the mechanism by which obesity associates with a given pathology is unknown or, in any case, not well established. Potential influences, not thoroughly investigated, include diet (quantitative? qualitative?), endocrine status (leptin? estrogens?), heredity, metabolic features (dyslipidemia? increased blood glucose?), fitness, additional comorbidities and age of onset of obesity.

PATHOLOGY	COMMENT	REFERENCE
All-cancer mortality enhanced, men and women	Cohort	[352]
Breast cancer risk enhanced, postmenopausal women	Cohort	[353]
Prostate cancer mortality enhanced	Cohort	[354]
Colon cancer risk enhanced, men and women	Cohort	[355]
Colon cancer prognosis worsened, men and women	Cohort	[356]
Colon cancer mortality enhanced, men and women	Cohort	[357]
Renal-cell carcinoma risk enhanced, men and women	Correlative, case-control	[358]
Endometrial carcinoma risk enhanced	Cohort	[359]
Gallstones risk enhanced, women	Cohort	[360]
Pregnancy complications risk enhanced	Cohort	[361]
Dementia in middle-aged men risk enhanced	Cohort	[362]
Dementia-of-elderly risk enhanced, women	Cohort	[363]
Dementia risk enhanced	Cohort	[364]
Postoperative wound infection risk enhanced	Cohort	[365]
Knee osteoarthritis risk enhanced, men and women	Cohort	[366]
Esophagitis risk enhanced, men and women	Correlative, case-control	[367]
Risk of hypoventilation	Correlative, case-control	[368]
Obstructive sleep apnea risk enhanced, men and women	Cohort	[369]
Urinary incontinence risk enhanced, women	Cohort	[370]
Fetal defects risk enhanced	Cohort	[371]

PATHOLOGY	COMMENT	REFERENCE
Heart failure risk enhanced	Cohort	[372]
False positive mammography risk enhanced	Correlative	[373]
Gout risk enhanced	Cohort	[374]
Stroke risk enhanced in men	Cohort	[375]
Kidney stone risk enhanced	Cohort	[376]
Fatty liver disease risk enhanced	Correlative	[377]

THE METABOLIC SYNDROME

Although the health-related associations with obesity described above are important, a principal focus of public health interest has been on a somewhat loosely defined entity called the metabolic syndrome (see **APPENDIX 2**). The diagnosis is to be made when any three or more of the following factors are present [378]:

1. Waist circumference exceeding 40 inches (102 cm) for men and 35 inches (88 cm) for women.
2. Fasting blood triglyceride concentration (a typical species of fat found in blood) exceeding 150 mg/dL.
3. Fasting blood HDL-cholesterol (good cholesterol) less than 40 mg/dL for men and less than 50 mg/dL for women
4. Blood pressure exceeding 130 systolic and 85 diastolic (hypertension)
5. Fasting blood glucose concentration exceeding 110 mg/dL (diabetes mellitus type II or diabetic tendency).

Concern has been expressed about the waist measurement. An international consortium has recommended different cutoff points for different ethnic/regional populations. The value above is recommended for Americans and persons of European ancestry. Values for other populations have been published [379].

The reason for the intensity of interest in this syndrome is its close association with cardiovascular disease, heart attacks, strokes and gangrene of the lower extremities. A survey of a large representative group of adult Americans conducted in 2003 revealed that the syndrome was present in 22.8% of adult men and 22.6% of adult women. The prevalence was 4.6% in normal weight (BMI less than 25) persons, 22.4% in overweight (BMI 25-29.9) persons, and 59.6% in obese (BMI 30 or more) persons [380]. Aging is associated with a progressive increase in prevalence. In a representative sampling of American adults, both genders included, prevalence was 6.7% in persons aged 20 to 29 years and 43.5% in persons aged 60 to 69 years in 2002 [381]. In a population of children aged 4 to 20 years, of mixed white, black and Hispanic origins, there was prevalence of a modified definition of metabolic syndrome, believed appropriate for children, of 38.7% in moderately obese children and 49.7% in severely obese subjects in 2004. The metabolic syndrome was absent in nonobese and overweight children. Classification for obesity was by BMI adapted for children [382].

In both men and women the presence of the metabolic syndrome is significantly associated with all cause mortality, cardiovascular mortality and the presence of cardiovascular disease [383-387]. There is evidence that cardiorespiratory fitness reduces the risk of both all-cause mortality and cardiovascular mortality in men with the metabolic syndrome [385;388]. As the population of industrialized countries ages, if the prevalence of metabolic syndrome increases, painful adjustments in the delivery of medical care may be necessitated by intolerable costs [389].

The factors listed above constitute a statistical cluster i.e. the presence of any factor is associated with increased likelihood of the presence of one or more of the other factors [390]. There is interest in refining the definition of this syndrome in order more accurately to focus attention on persons most at risk, to increase the sensitivity and specificity for cardiovascular disease screening. Suggestions have included additional chemical measurements and modifications of the above measurements (see **Metabolic Syndrome** in **APPENDIX 2**). The syndrome as defined above is a rather crude idea. The separate components are given equal weight in this formulation although they probably are not of equal predictive value. It is not clear which combinations of components provide greater risk than others. Treatment may be directed to each separate component which is present. There is no treatment for the syndrome, *per se*, [391] other than weight loss which improves all components.

Two subgroups of persons who probably should have more attention than they have received are the metabolically obese normal weight persons and the metabolically healthy obese persons [392]. Metabolically obese normal weight persons are not obese as defined by BMI but have the metabolic syndrome and, specifically, increased visceral adipose tissue. The prevalence of this subgroup in the general population has not been well established. In a population aged 70 to 79 years, Goodpaster and colleagues [393] found a prevalence of the metabolic syndrome of 12% in "normal weight" (BMI) men and 22% in "normal weight" women. Some metabolically obese normal weight persons are young and their age and absence of obesity may result in their not being recognized until a cardiovascular or other consequence signals their risk status. Metabolically healthy but obese persons do not have the risk factors of the metabolic syndrome but are obese as defined by BMI. They may account for as much as 20% of the obese population. Aggressive treatment of them may not be justified [394].

At least some of the difficulty in evaluating this group may be the result of reliance on the BMI to assess adiposity. Another possibility is suggested by the finding in chickens, mice and monkeys that infection with a certain virus (human adenovirus-36) frequently infecting humans produces a syndrome characterized by obesity and lowered blood cholesterol and triglycerides. The presence of antibodies to the virus in humans, indicating infection at some time, is associated with obesity and lowered blood cholesterol and triglycerides [395].

Waist circumference is assumed to be a surrogate for visceral adipose tissue and is an obvious target for substitution by something better. However, it is easily measured, readily available, inexpensive and consequently useful and frequently used. The value for thresholds for concern, the cutoff points, mentioned above, 40 in. (102 cm.) for men and 35 in. (88 cm.) for women are not derived from risk factors but are derived from a chosen BMI, 30 for both men and women. The cutoff points identify men and women more likely than not to have a BMI of 30 or more in a randomly selected group of residents of north Glasgow, Scotland [396]. There is circularity in this concept which suggests the thought that more research and better indices are needed. A large study of a representative sample of American white adults of both genders showed that waist circumference has a closer statistical association with cardiovascular risk factors than does BMI [397]. Possibly the risk of any given waist circumference is dependent on age and ethnicity/race.

When American subjects are classified by BMI, normal 18.5-24.9, overweight 25.0-29.9, obese 30.-34.9, prevalence of the metabolic syndrome increases as BMI increases. However, within each BMI classification a waist circumference exceeding 40 in (102 cm) for men and 35 in (88 cm) for women was associated with a greater prevalence of one or more of the metabolic variables of the syndrome, hypertension, dyslipidemia and diabetes mellitus type II [398]. Regardless of the presence or absence of obesity and regardless of the degree of adiposity, the presence of a large waist circumference is associated with a greater prevalence of the metabolic syndrome and, consequently, a greater risk of cardiovascular disease.

A troubling finding has been an increase in waist circumference disproportionate to the increase in BMI in American children [399]. In children waist circumference is a good index of visceral adipose tissue estimated by magnetic resonance imaging [400].

The metabolic syndrome is a critically important entity. Multiple large prospective studies indicate that the presence of at least three elements of the syndrome confers an approximately two-fold increase in the risk of death, heart attack, stroke, or heart failure. As the number of elements of the syndrome present increases, the risk of cardiovascular disease and specifically coronary heart disease increases to four-fold to six-fold[386;390;401-403]. Increased visceral adipose tissue, together with associated elements of the metabolic syndrome, is also a risk factor for development of dementia [404]. There is evidence that obesity, *per se*, is associated with cognitive decline, independently from diabetes [405]. Consistent with that finding is the demonstration that higher BMI is associated with atrophy in various sites in the brain independently of diabetes in cognitively normal elderly obese and overweight persons. The authors were of the opinion that excess adiposity was the indirect source of the changes in brain structure rather than the reverse. A valuable experiment would be an attempt to demonstrate a reversal of the brain alterations by weight loss [406].

What are the mechanisms by which waist circumference is related to development of the metabolic risk factors? Current belief is that large waist circumference indicates a large deposit of intraabdominal, visceral, adipose tissue which alters liver metabolism toward development of the lipid, glucose, and blood pressure components of the metabolic syndrome. Although measurement of waist circumference has provided important and useful results in epidemiological surveys as a measure of visceral fat it is obviously only an approximation. It cannot distinguish between intraabdominal fat and subcutaneous abdominal fat. There can be difficulties about where to measure it. Should it be the largest abdominal circumference? Should it be halfway between the lower rib margin and the upper brim of the pelvis, as many have advocated? Some have recommended measurement at the level of the umbilicus. In that case, what about large pendulous abdomens in which the umbilicus may be lower than the pelvic brim? A clinical manual published by the American Medical Association recommends that the measurement be made at the upper level of the pelvic brim, parallel to floor with the patient standing,[407]. It seems, *a priori*, that if the hypothesis that development of the metabolic syndrome is a manifestation of the amount of visceral adipose tissue that a more direct estimate of the amount of visceral adipose tissue would be desirable.

Visceral adipose tissue has been estimated by computer assisted tomography (CAT scan), by magnetic resonance imaging (MRI scan), and by ultrasound imaging. There has been a tendency to adopt computerized tomography as the method of choice. The machines are widely available. Many studies have shown acceptable reproducibility [408]. Cut off points correlated with likelihood of cardiovascular risk factors have been documented [409]. The most frequently performed procedure is measurement of the area of intraabdominal adipose tissue displayed in a single cross-sectional image taken between the fourth and fifth lumbar vertebrae. Estimation of adipose tissue in the cross section has been validated by correlation with planimetry of the same cross sections in band-sawed cadavers [410] Results in surveys correlate statistically with cardiovascular risk factors. However, there is evidence that for evaluation of single individuals a better procedure might be multiple serial images in the lumbar region and calculation of the volume of adipose tissue [411-413]. Multiple images increase exposure to X-rays, an important consideration in research surveys, especially of children.

An advantage of magnetic resonance imaging is that there is no exposure to X-rays. Results have been generally similar to comparable computerized tomography examinations. Reproducibility has been acceptable. However, there is clear evidence that a single image may not correctly index the findings of multiple serial images for visceral adipose tissue. [414]. Estimation of measurement of adipose tissue by magnetic resonance imaging has been validated by dissection in pigs [415] and three human cadavers [416]. Measurements of visceral adipose tissue by magnetic resonance imaging seem to be well correlated with elements of the metabolic syndrome [417].

Visceral adipose tissue can be indexed ultrasonographically by measuring the distance between the posterior surface of the anterior abdominal wall and the anterior surface of the lumbar spine. This index correlates well with waist circumference, and with the single-image computerized tomography procedure. Reproducibility is good [418]. Correlations with elements of the metabolic syndrome are significant and better than with waist circumference [419].

A sometimes overlooked distinction is that the imaging techniques index the volume of adipose tissue, not the mass of fat. Adipose tissue consists of adipocytes, water, and a variety of cells of diverse origin, especially macrophages, cells of the immune system. Martin and colleagues dissected the adipose tissue from six unembalmed male cadavers and found, by densitometric technique, that the lipid fraction ranged from 0.54 to 0.85 [420]. It is possible that the metabolic syndrome is better correlated with the volume of adipose tissue than the quantity of fat.

In congenital generalized lipodystrophy, a rare genetically mediated disorder in which adipose tissue is nearly absent, there is markedly fatty liver and there are elements of the metabolic syndrome [421;422]. In surveys of obese and overweight persons in whom fat in liver was indexed by biopsy, elements of the metabolic syndrome were associated with fatty liver [421;423;424].

The venous drainage of the visceral fat goes directly to the liver before reaching the heart and lungs, in contrast to fat located subcutaneously and elsewhere for which the venous drainage goes to the heart and lungs. Danforth [112] suggested that when adipose tissues are unable readily to accept fat deposits the excess fat is deposited in liver. This idea has been the basis of the "overflow hypothesis" [421]. According to this hypothesis, when products of fat metabolism cannot be accommodated by adipose tissue, especially visceral adipose tissue, they will be lodged in liver where they mediate the glucose and lipid abnormalities of the metabolic syndrome, elevated fasting blood glucose, elevated fasting blood triglyceride, and depressed HDL cholesterol, resulting in enhanced risk of cardiovascular disease.

While this mechanism probably contributes significantly to features of the metabolic syndrome principal emphasis has shifted to the role of adipocytokines [425]. An adipocytokine is a hormone secreted by cells of the adipose tissue. The responsible cells are adipocytes, "fat cells", and macrophages, "inflammatory cells", part of the immune system. A long list of hormones of somewhat uncertain significance are produced: leptin, described above in detail, adiponectin, tumor necrosis factor-α, interleukin-1, interleukin-6, retinol binding protein-4, visfatin, resistin and others. On the basis of experiments with laboratory animals and data obtained in clinical investigations a picture is beginning to emerge in which adipocytokines as a system are a link between obesity and the morbidities type II diabetes mellitus, the metabolic syndrome, cardiovascular disease and certain cancers [426;427].

ADIPOCYTOKINES

Some of the important facts supporting this idea are found both in studies of experimental animals and in studies of humans. Production by adipose tissue of the adipocytkines tumor necrosis factor-α, interleukin-1, inrterleukin-6, resistin and leptin is associated with the metabolic syndrome [428]. Blood concentration of adiponectin is reduced in people with the metabolic syndrome [429].

The concentration of leptin in blood is increased in obesity and decreases with weight loss. In contrast the concentration of adiponectin is *decreased* in obesity and *increases* with weight loss whether mediated by surgery [430] or by diet [431]. The increase in adiponectin is closely related to decrease in visceral adipose tissue. See Visceral Obesity above. In mice experimentally manipulated to produce models of obesity and diabetes, administration of adiponectin reduced insulin resistance, the core metabolic defect in type II diabetes [432] (see **Diabetes** in **APPENDIX 2**). Administration of tumor necrosis factor-α reduced production of adiponectin in mice and increased insulin resistance [433]. Both tumor necrosis factor-α and interleukin 6 are increased in the blood by obesity and reduced by weight loss [434;435], especially loss of visceral fat [430].

Tumor necrosis factor-α and interleukin-6 provide a mechanism by which increased adipose tissue enhances insulin resistance and consequently causes diabetes mellitus type II. Adiponectin provides a mechanism by which weight loss, reducing tumor necrosis factor-α and interleukin-6, can reduce insulin resistance. In addition to this reciprocal relationship, adiponectin can ameliorate insulin resistance directly by pathways not involving tumor necrosis factor-α and interleukin-6. Likewise, tumor necrosis factor-α and interleukin-6 can exacerbate insulin resistance by pathways not involving adiponectin.

Analogously, adiponectin opposes the processes producing cardiovascular disease and hypertension by its effects on arteries and the heart. The pathogenic effects are enhanced by tumor necrosis factor-α and interleukin-6.

The critical role of the intraabdominal fat in the mediation of the above mechanisms associated with risk of cardiovascular disease is demonstrated by reports that liposuction, surgical removal, of large amounts of subcutaneous fat from abdomen, arms, flanks, hips, and thighs does not alter risk factors, blood pressure, blood glucose, insulin resistance, cholesterol and triglycerides and does not alter blood adiponectin, tumor necrosis factor-α, and interleukin-6. Leptin was reduced and the amount of weight lost was representative of the amounts of weight lost by diet and exercise which do improve the profile of risk factors for cardiovascular disease [436].

The arrow diagram (Figure 4) is a model of the activities of the principal adipocytokines, tumor necrosis factor-α, and adiponectin, as presently understood. Tumor necrosis factor-α enhances mechanisms promoting cardiovascular disease and the principal feature of diabetes mellitus type II, insulin resistance. It also inhibits production of adiponectin which defends against cardiovascular disease and diabetes mellitus type II and also inhibits production of tumor necrosis factor-α.

Present understanding of this system depends significantly on results of experiments with rodent model systems and may be modified by ongoing clinical investigations [437-440]

The adipocytokine system, seen as a link between obesity and disease, offers several inviting targets for drug-based intervention, especially adiponectin. There is much ongoing research directed to discovery of a new therapy. It would be ironic if a way is found to prevent disease without weight loss and its painful requirements [441]

Obesity, especially visceral obesity, has been claimed to be a risk factor for many cancers, especially cancer of breast, endometrium, prostate, gall bladder, colon and stomach. No mechanism for this effect has been established and it may vary by site and type of the malignancy. It has been suggested that cancer risk is enhanced by the characteristic alteration of secretion of adipocytokines in obesity, increased leptin and interleukin-6 and decreased secretion of adiponectin [442].

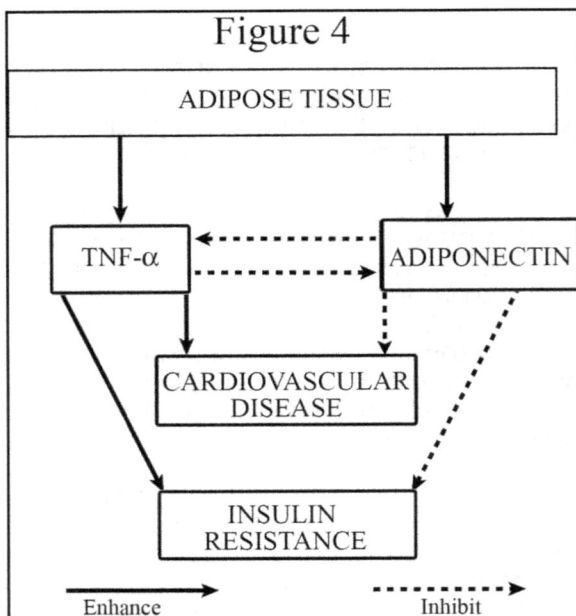

Figure 4

ADIPOSE TISSUE

TNF-α

ADIPONECTIN

CARDIOVASCULAR DISEASE

INSULIN RESISTANCE

Enhance

Inhibit

CHAPTER FIVE: TREATMENT

There are three general categories of measures designed to remedy, and sometimes to prevent, obesity. They are: 1) conventional, i.e. usual care; 2) surgical; and 3) public health measures.

USUAL CARE

This therapeutic modality includes nearly always a diet prescription, usually a prescription for exercise, frequently a prescription of drugs, and sometimes a program of behavior modification. The diet prescription and exercise prescription range in intensity and formality from an incidental advice, "you should lose some weight, get more exercise, eat less", to highly structured programs characterized by detailed planning and monitoring.

There has long been agreement that weight loss, achieved by usual care, of 10% or even less, of body weight by obese persons with cardiovascular risk factors is followed by easily demonstrable improvements in hypertension, blood cholesterol values, blood triglycerides and blood glucose of diabetics [443]. Furthermore, it has been shown that sustained weight loss of 15 pounds (6.8 kg) by overweight and obese persons (BMI exceeding 24.9), middle aged and older, having normal blood pressure, substantially reduced the long-term risk of developing hypertension [444]. It has been shown that modest sustained, but not nonsustained, weight loss reduces the risk of developing diabetes mellitus type II, formerly called noninsulin-dependent diabetes mellitus. Sustained but not nonsustained weight loss maintained reduced blood pressure and other risk factors for coronary heart disease [445]. In a controlled study of nondiabetic obese men (BMI 30 or more) with erectile dysfunction who lost 10% or more body weight by a regime of diet and exercise one third of the subjects experienced improved erectile function while the weight-stable control group experienced no improvement [446]. Weight loss mediated by diet and exercise reduces symptoms of osteoarthritis of the knee [447] in over weight and obese persons. Loss of 10% of body weight significantly reduced symptoms of obstructive sleep apnea [219]. Weight loss reduces the risk of gout [374].

It is likely that much of the metabolic benefit is attributable to reduction of visceral fat. There is evidence that reduction of visceral fat more effectively reduces components of the metabolic syndrome (see **Metabolic Syndrome** in **APPENDIX 2**), than does reduction of subcutaneous fat [448] and persons with abundant visceral fat tend to lose visceral fat preferentially, at least initially, during diet-induced weight loss [449].

Given the above well-accepted short term benefits it seems that it should be easily possible to demonstrate that weight loss reduces mortality. This issue has been the subject of serious research efforts since 1951 [450]. There have been reports that weight loss by overweight or obese persons *increases* mortality [321;451-457], *has no influence* on mortality [456;458] or *reduces* mortality [459-462] . The studies cited differ from each other in significant ways. They are cited not so much to demonstrate conflicts of data but rather to demonstrate that differing ways of approaching the same difficult question, what is the effect of weight loss on mortality, can lead to different conclusions. All are epidemiological surveys in which a population of interest is surveyed at one time and then, with no intervention, survivors are surveyed at another time. Features to be surveyed are indicated by the following series of questions: Was weight loss intentional or unintentional? Is it possible reliably to determine the difference [463]? What was the base line weight? What was the motive for losing weight? How much weight was lost, if any? Are the data self-reported or measured? By what means was weight lost? Was weight loss sustained or fluctuating [464]? Were tobacco or alcohol use possible factors? Were comorbidities diabetes mellitus type II, hypertension, cardiovascular disease and cancer at base line accounted for? What was the cause of death? Obviously age and gender must be considered [465-467] .These confounding factors make it extremely difficult to perform a convincing epidemiological study. The ideal approach to questions of this sort is the clinical trials model. In such a study a large representative sample of the population of interest is recruited, base line data are obtained by valid means, and the sample is randomly divided into two groups, control and intervention. One half is required to lose a prescribed amount of weight by a prescribed means. The other half is not encouraged to attempt to lose weight. After a suitable time, many years, the survivors are counted, relevant measures performed, and the causes of death in those who did not survive determined. Obviously this study, the clinical trial model, cannot be performed and it cannot be conclusively stated that intentional weight loss has an adverse influence on longevity.

Numerous studies have demonstrated that patients with established chronic heart failure who are overweight or obese, based on BMI, have lower all cause and cardiovascular mortality than lean people with established chronic heart failure [468]. This has been called the "obesity paradox" because obesity and overweight are important risk factors for the incidence of cardiovascular disease generally and for enhanced mortality [469]. The mechanism for the paradox is unknown. Understanding is made difficult by the existence of a wasting syndrome called "cardiac cachexia". There is some inconclusive evidence that diet-induced weight loss is beneficial for obese and overweight patients with established heart failure [470]. However, a program to lose weight should be undertaken with caution.

A study of elderly men with long followup found that men who became overweight in midlife and then lost weight in late life were at greater risk for cardiovascular disease and mortality than men who had constant normal weight or constant overweight through decades of life. Was weight loss intentional and if so what was the motive [471]?

A reason for thinking that weight loss might extend longevity is found in experiments showing that restriction of caloric intake increases longevity in laboratory organisms, yeast, flies, worms, mice and monkeys. In a 20 year randomized, controlled study of monkeys, restriction of caloric intake by 30% delayed onset of age-related death, diabetes, cardiovascular disease, cancer and brain atrophy [472]. There are few humans who would willingly tolerate a lifetime 30% restriction of caloric intake. However there is suggestive evidence that the findings in monkeys would be duplicated in humans if the experiment were performed [473-475]. Restriction of caloric intake is a feature of almost every weight reduction regimen.

What do these facts mean for people contemplating weight reduction and their advisers? The emphasis should be on comorbidities and the risk of comorbidities. Any person, obese or overweight, with diabetes mellitus type II, hypertension, or the metabolic syndrome will quickly benefit from weight loss. Blood pressure, blood glucose, blood cholesterol and blood triglycerides are rapidly reduced. Frankly obese persons, usually defined as having a BMI 30 or greater, are at high risk for multiple comorbidities. As described above, some investigators believe that possibly intentional weight loss can be associated with a long term reduction of longevity. Not everyone believes that. Even so the risk to benefit ratio could be favorable if benefit includes quality of life.

Since the middle of the twentieth century there has been concern that weight reduction by dieting may be a cause of depression [476]. This concern has faded with time and empirical studies have not demonstrated an association of depression with dieting for weight loss [477].

There is an association, by definition, of dieting for weight loss and the eating disorders anorexia nervosa and bulimia nervosa, since diagnostic criteria for both disorders include voluntary restriction of caloric intake and weight loss [478]. For a description of these diagnostic categories see **Eating Disorders** in **APPENDIX 2**.

Young women who develop eating disorders often have a history of dieting and it has been suggested that dieting plays an etiologic role in the development of eating disorders. A prospective study of 15 year old London school girls revealed an eight-fold relative risk of developing an eating disorder in the girls who dieted [479]. Interviews of 2,163 female twins revealed a concordance rate for bulimia of 22.9% in identical twins and 8.7% in fraternal twins. Numerous epidemiologic factors, and comorbid psychopathology, were assessed. The data were interpreted as showing that development of bulimia nervosa "is substantially influenced by both epidemiologic and genetic risk factors" [480]. Three prospective, controlled studies have demonstrated no increase in symptoms of eating disorders following weight loss mediated by caloric restriction [481-483]. It seems likely that dieting is a manifestation, a symptom, of eating disorders instead of a cause [484;485].

A very large number of people in industrialized societies have in recent years been subject to fluctuations of weight, weight cycling by weight loss followed by weight regain, frequently multiple times, as a consequence of a weight loss program followed by failure to maintain the weight loss. There has long been concern that such cycling may be associated with increased morbidity and mortality, especially from coronary heart disease. Numerous studies have been reported, none definitive, and frequently presenting conflicting conclusions. This is an extremely difficult subject to study. The clinical trial model, described above in the paragraphs discussing the possible influence of weight loss on mortality, cannot be utilized. Questions to be considered in experimental design are: What is the weight at the initiation of cycling? How is "cycling" defined? How is cycling to be expressed numerically for statistical purposes? How many data points are needed? At what intervals? How many repetitions of cycling are significant? At what velocity? Was weight loss intentional or unintentional? How is preexisting disease to be considered? How must alcohol and tobacco use be considered? How long must the followup be? How are the data to be obtained? Even if a clinical trial were possible, as a practical matter, and an association of morbidity and mortality with weight cycling were demonstrated there would remain the critically important question: By what biological mechanism is the association mediated?

Two mechanisms have been proposed but not established. Firstly, there is evidence that weight loss results in increased concentrations of organochlorine pollutants in blood and subcutaneous adipose tissue [486]. Organochlorine pollutants are environmental pollutants of agricultural and industrial origins which are widely distributed in the environment and are found in the tissues of many fish, birds, and mammals in many parts of the world [487]. It has been suspected that they may play an etiological role in several kinds of cancer and an assortment of other ailments [488]. Secondly, there is some evidence that weight loss and regain promotes abdominal adiposity, a component of the metabolic syndrome [489]. However, the consensus seems to be that, despite some inconclusive conflicting data, weight cycling in the absence of preexisting disease and known risk factors is not harmful [490]

Concern has been expressed about the composition of weight lost by dieting. When the fraction of weight lost as fat by 7 obese dieting women was measured by 5 of the methods described in Chapter Two, entitled "How is Obesity Measured?". The values for percent of weight loss as fat ranged from 87% to 91.5% with an average weight loss of 31 lb. (14 kg) [491]. This seems intuitively to be a physiologically acceptable outcome since loss of fat would necessarily obligate some loss of fat-free mass, especially water. The diet used was a commercially available liquid diet.

There is no doubt that obese persons who experience rapid, large losses of weight achieved by gastrointestinal surgery or very low Calorie diets (300 to 800 Calories/day) are at significantly greater risk of gallstone formation than obese persons of stable weight. Obese persons whose weight is stable are at greater risk for gallstones than normal weight persons whose weight is stable. Weight-loss associated gallstones are often asymptomatic, as are any gallstones, and will sometimes disappear with no intervention [492]. Data suggest that rates of weight loss less than 3.3 lbs./week (1.5 kg.) do not enhance risk of gall stone formation [493].

Intentional weight loss in both older women [494] and older men [495] results in reduced bone mineral density. In older women,[496] and probably in older men,[497] there is increased risk of hip fracture. There is evidence that calcium supplementation of the diet minimizes bone loss during caloric restriction [494] in older women. Clinicians prescribing Calorie restricted diets for older people may want to consider also prescribing measures protective of bone, calcium, vitamin D, exercise, or drugs. In a one year randomized controlled trial intentional diet-mediated weight loss of an average 10% of body weight resulted in reduced bone mineral density of the hip despite dietary counseling, calcium and vitamin D supplementation and a program of vigorous exercise [498]. Caution is advisable.

Conventional Diet

There is a huge mass of publications concerning weight-reduction/weight-maintenance diets both in professional journals and in the lay press. Searching Amazon in 2006 for "weight loss" revealed

2,590 books. A detailed review from a scientific perspective of some of the popular diets described in most of these books has been published [499]. Evaluations were generally unfavorable.

Persons who recognize that a tendency to deposit excessive body fat will endure for life will be disappointed in the professional literature for the reason that evaluation of the merits and possible adverse consequences of the diets described encompasses, in most instances, intervals of only weeks or months. A small number of reports of experimental interventions describe results obtained during one to five years. What we need to know is what the merits and possible adverse consequences are during intervals of decades. Valuable insights have come from survey studies of national and ethnic populations in which adherence to traditional diets is presumably of life-long duration [500-502].

There are controversies about what constitutes an appropriate weight loss or weight maintenance diet, especially concerning the fat content [503]. How much fat? Which fats? These controversies tend to obscure the fact that there is broad consensus concerning the appropriate characteristics of weight-reduction/weight-maintenance diets among a very large majority of professionals, scholars, clinicians of every kind, researchers. A listing of those characteristics may seem forbidding to a person seeking practical advice about a weight-reduction/weight-maintenance diet. However, there are many practical aids. An excellent one is *Dietary Guidelines for Americans*, published by the U.S. Department of Health and Human Services, available free online at: *www.healthierus.gov/ dietaryguidelines* (accessed 02/23/2010). Printed copies can be purchased by calling toll-free (866) 512 1800. This publication can be supplemented by an offering of the US Department of Agriculture called *MyPyramid* available at *http://mypyramid.gov/* (accessed 02/23/2010). Use of these guides, providing detailed advice about food, using household measures, will allow easy design of meals consistent with the consensus.

Dietary characteristics about which there is consensus are:

•The caloric value of the diet must be sufficiently low to bring about the desired weight loss, in the instance of a weight loss regimen, and sufficiently low to maintain the target weight, in the instance of a weight maintenance regimen. No amount of juggling the qualitative composition of the diet will allow escape from this quantitative fact. The amount of weight lost over periods of time of interest will be proportional to the caloric deficit incurred. Alteration of the protein/carbohydrate/fat composition of the diet, within a broad range will enhance weight loss only to the extent that it enhances caloric deficit [504;505]. Freedom to alter the composition of the diet allows for the design of highly individualized programs. This is important because the weight-maintenance program must be continued for life, with some revision from time to time to account for changed circumstances.

•There must be sufficient protein of sufficient biological value to maintain bodily integrity and to supply an adequate quantity of the eight amino acids which humans cannot synthesize (see **Amino Acids** in **APPENDIX 2**).

•Fat intake, analogous to protein intake, must have adequate quantities of two polyunsaturated fatty acids, alpha-linolenic and linoleic acid, which cannot be synthesized by the human body and must be obtained from dietary sources. The saturated fatty acids known as trans fatty acids and the cholesterol should be as low as possible [506].

•Dietary fiber is nondigestable carbohydrate from plant foods. It reduces risk of heart disease, improves bowel function and may reduce risk of some cancers. Few Americans get recommended amounts, 38 and 25 g/day for men and women respectively.

•There must be adequate intake of the minerals sodium, potassium, calcium, iron and magnesium.

•Attention must be given to intake of vitamins A, B, C, D and E. Healthy people will get adequate amounts from an appropriate diet but special circumstances may require supplementation, e.g. pregnancy.

•Alcoholic beverages should not exceed two drinks daily.

Low Carbohydrate, High Protein, High Fat Diets

In 1972 Dr. Robert Atkins published a description of a low carbohydrate, high protein diet, *Dr. Atkins' Diet Revolution*, which sold 15 million copies. In 1992 he published *Dr. Atkins' New Diet Revolution* which was on the New York Times best-seller list for seven years and inspired numerous imitations and modifications. The Atkins diet has been considered the model for low carbohydrate, high protein diets. In 1989 Dr. Atkins founded the company Atkins Nutritionals to market products prominent in the diet described in the books. After an initial rapid success, sales declined steeply in the year 2004 and the company declared bankruptcy in August, 2005. In April, 2003 Dr. Atkins died following a fall.

There have been at least four randomized trials of one year duration in which low carbohydrate, high protein diets were compared with a variety of other popular diets [507-510]. Among these studies there have been differences of diet composition, and in the subjects of age, gender, initial weight and comorbidities. All have been plagued by large dropout rates, diminishing adherence and the necessity of relying on self reported adherence.

Diets employed have been Atkins (low carbohydrate, high protein), Ornish (very low fat), Zone (reduced fat, conventional), Weight Watchers (reduced fat, conventional), LEARN (reduced fat, conventional) and other low fat, conventional diets. After *6 months* all tested diets were associated with significant weight loss, more with the low carbohydrate diet in three of the four trials [508-510]. After *one year* only one of the four studies revealed greater weight loss for the low carbohydrate diet [509]. In three of four studies there was some regain at one year from the 6 months value for all diets [508-510]. For all diets in all studies weight loss at one year was of the order of 3-5%. There were scattered slight improvements in risk factors for cardiovascular disease, blood pressure, and dyslipidemia. No diet in any study was associated with a significant worsening of risk factors, a surprising finding in the instance of the Atkins diet.

There has been interest in the reasons for the initially somewhat greater weight loss frequently observed for low carbohydrate diets versus low fat diets. Suggestions have included a greater reduction of caloric intake in persons taking the low carbohydrate diet as a consequence of a greater satiating effect of that diet and/or as a consequence of relative absence of variety in the menu of the low carbohydrate diet. Some commercial low carbohydrate diet products lack palatability [511]. An additional mechanism described by Feinman and Fine [512] is the result of the ability of low carbohydrate intake to stimulate conversion of dietary protein to glucose [513]. The conversion introduces inefficiency of 25-30% in the metabolism of protein [514]. The "lost" Calories are expected to be in the form of heat manifested as increased thermic effect of food (see *Energetics* in Chapter Three). Indeed, Johnston *et al.* demonstrated increased thermic effect of the food of a popular high protein diet compared with that of a conventional high carbohydrate, low fat diet [515]. The greater thermic effect of protein food compared with carbohydrate foods is well established and long known [516-519].

Few experts would recommend long maintenance on a low carbohydrate, high protein diet. Reasons include the absence of long term data on either efficacy or safety [520]. Specific concerns are the tendency to calcium loss in urine and consequent risk of bone loss and occurrence of kidney stones [521] and some evidence that high protein diets cause progression of existing coronary artery heart disease [522] in people following such diets. There is some inconclusive evidence that low carbohydrate, high fat diets impair cognitive function [523;524].

Very Low Calorie Diets

Diets providing fewer than 800 Calories per day are called very low Calorie diets. They should be employed seldom, for unusual reasons, for only a few months, with intensive medical supervision, and often with supplementation with minerals, and vitamins. In the decade before 1983 at least 60 deaths were attributed to such regimens. Apparently safety can be assured by appropriate choice of the protein and carbohydrate components and vitamin and mineral supplementation [525;526]. However such diets alone are no better than other forms of obesity treatment in achieving the critically important goal of habituation to a lifetime of weight-control practices [527].

Mediterranean Diet

The traditional Mediterranean diet is different from a typical American diet in its higher content of fruits, vegetables, legumes, fish and monounsaturated fats as olive oil. It is lower in meat and poultry and includes regular but moderate intake of wine and lower intake of dairy products. There has been interest in a reduced-Calorie version for weight loss because there is evidence that it may be protective of the heart [528]. Few data concerning weight loss are presently available but the diet may ultimately be a good alternative to the conventional low fat diet.

Exercise

Usual care often includes an element of exercise prescription ranging from casual advice to "get more exercise" to an enrollment in a formal program. Exercise confers many benefits, reduced risk of heart disease, reduced risk of diabetes mellitus type II, improved blood pressure, and improved mood and appearance. These features are important but will not be reviewed because the focus of this text is on weight loss, and weight maintenance.

Exercise would seem a peculiarly appropriate treatment for treatment of obesity because expenditure of the energy, Calories, ingested as food can contribute to the energy deficit required for weight loss. Vigorous exercise suppresses appetite for intervals of several hours to several days [529]. During moderate exercise obese men obtain a greater proportion of energy from fat than do lean men [530]. A study of female twins showed that physical activity does not have a lesser effect on body fat mass in persons with a genetic predisposition to obesity [531]. There is clear evidence that obese men can achieve substantial losses of weight and of body fat by exercise without reduction of caloric intake [532]. However, the consensus seems to be that, as a practical matter, exercise should be regarded as an adjunct to diet and not a principal device for achieving weight loss. This is not surprising. The attrition rate in exercise programs is high. Under conditions of life in industrialized societies few people are required to experience much physical exertion. Machines do the heavy lifting. The automobile has eliminated need for much walking. Asking people to exercise is asking them to experience what our ancestors strived to make it possible for us to avoid.

What kind of exercise should be chosen? How much exercise should be accomplished?

From the perspective of weight loss the essential feature is the caloric expenditure. From the perspective of weight maintenance regular performance for an indefinite period of time is an essential feature. Fortunately there are many possibilities. The appropriate choice requires consideration of the level of caloric expenditure, personal interest and taste, the practical possibilities, and the stage of life. Whatever is chosen must be done regularly for as long as it is appropriate. In youth perhaps it will be running, in middle life walking, and in advanced age stretching exercises. People with medical disabilities, cardiac, musculoskeletal, neurological, metabolic or other, should consult a physician before undertaking an exercise program. Some people may choose to enroll in a formal program offered by a medical center. Fitness centers often have personnel qualified to give advice. An excellent source of information about getting started is the government publication, 2008 Physical Activity Guidelines for Americans, published by the US Department of Health and Human Service: *http://www.health.gov/paguidelines/guidelines/default.aspx* (Accessed 2/24/10). The guidelines reflect approximate consensus, derived from extensive data, concerning how much exercise is desirable for general health maintenance and for weight maintenance. The recommendation is that adults, in the absence of contraindications, should have at least 150 minutes of moderate intensity exercise per week or at least 75 minutes of vigorous intensity exercise per week. The report gives numerous examples of vigorous activity and of moderate activity.

There is a clear relation between the amount/intensity of exercise and weight loss, i.e. a dose-response relationship. Consequently persons seeking weight loss may need to engage in more and more intense exercise [533] and persons previously obese who have achieved nonobese status, may also need more exercise for weight maintenance [534] The use of home exercise equipment may enhance adherence and weight loss [535]. Prolonged vigorous activity has the advantage that it results in significant increase in metabolic rate persisting more than 2 hours after cessation of exercise [536]. This is possible only for physically fit persons.

Some examples of moderate activity are walking at 3 miles per hour, social dancing, golf carrying the clubs, downhill skiing, gardening and yard work and home repairs. Some examples of vigorous activity are jogging, calisthenics, singles tennis, competitive football and basketball, cross-country skiing and shoveling heavy snow *http://www.cdc.gov/nccdphp/dnpa/physical/pdf/PA_Intensity_table_2_1.pdf* (accessed 02/25/10). Fitness centers with exercise machines can provide exercise of any desired intensity and type. Strength training is especially recommended for older adults to reduce the muscle deterioration which comes with age.

Drugs

No anti-obesity drugs are without "side effects", more properly called toxicities, sometimes serious. To be effective drugs will usually be taken for a long time. Available data do not establish their safety when taken for many years, perhaps decades. Sparse available data do not encourage hope that weight loss attributable to the drugs is maintained after withdrawal and often is not well maintained during continuation of drug ingestion [537-539]. Pharmacologic agents are to be used only in conjunction with programs of diet and exercise.

Attempts to use drugs to effect weight loss began more than a century ago with thyroid extract. In the modern era there has been transient enthusiasm for dinitrophenol, amphetamine, digitalis, diuretics, aminorex, fenfluramines, phenylpropanolamine, sibutramine and the herbal ephedra. All have been associated with unacceptable toxicities, in the instance of fenfluramine, lesions in valves of the heart. Fenfluramine and dexfenfluramine were withdrawn from the market in September 1997. Sibutramine was withdrawn from the market in October 2010 after demonstration that it enhanced the occurrence of heart attacks and strokes.

Only orlistat has been approved by the U.S. Food and Drug Administration for long term use. It is available without prescription. Phentermine, phendimetrazine, benzphetamine, and diethylpropion have been approved only for short term use, 12 weeks.

Orlistat modestly enhances weight loss induced by diet and exercise by preventing absorption of about 30% of ingested fat. The most frequent toxicities associated with orlistat have been loose oily stools, and frequent defecation The severity of this reaction is reduced by reducing the fat content of the diet [540]. Phentermine, phendimetrazine, benzphetamine and diethylpropion may cause rapid and irregular heart beat, insomnia, high blood pressure, dry mouth and constipation [541]. All of the approved drugs except orlistat are contraindicated in the presence of serious cardiovascular disease, including hypertension. There is no evidence that any of these agents improves mortality. Costs are significant [542].

The American College of Physicians has published clinical guidelines for use of pharmacological agents in the treatment of obesity [543]. Generally speaking, only frankly obese people conventionally defined as having a BMI of 30 or greater, are definitely candidates. This is the population in which the clearest, indisputable evidence of increased morbidity and mortality attributable to obesity has been found. Persons with a BMI of 25 to 30 and two or more obesity-related diseases or risk factors maybe considered under guidelines promulgated by the National Institutes of Health [314]. See the chapter entitled Medical Hazards of Obesity. A trial of diet, exercise, and life style changes only should be performed. If appropriate goals are not met pharmacological therapy may be considered for addition to the regimen. The patient should be fully informed of the risks and benefits of the agents and there must be careful medical supervision while they are being taken. The choice of agent should include consideration of the likely side effects for the individual patient and their acceptability [543].

There has been intense interest in medications for weight loss and much research seeking new and better agents [12]. Probably this has been dampened by discouraging failures of new agents to obtain regulatory approval. A new agent rimonabant has a novel mechanism of action. It suppresses appetite by blocking the same mechanism activated by the psychoactive agent of marijuana. However it seems to enhance suicide risk and is presently not approved for use anywhere after an initial experience with it in Europe.

Psychological Interventions

A variety of programs which might be called psychological interventions have been offered for the purposes of promoting weight loss and weight maintenance. They have been called behavior modification, lifestyle modification, cognitive therapy, psychotherapy, relaxation therapy and hypnotherapy. The most frequently provided and best-studied can be described as behavior modification, usually provided to groups of overweight people by dietitians or mental health professionals, usually as adjuncts to regimens of diet and exercise, sometimes with drugs. Characteristics of such programs have been described: "1) identifying eating or related life-style behaviors to be modified, 2) setting specific behavioral goals, 3) modifying determinants of the behavior to be changed, and 4) reinforcing the desired behavior. The goal of behavior treatment is to modify eating and physical activity habits, typically focusing on gradual changes" [544]. Methods employed include long-continued, regular contact between therapist and patient, self-monitoring of weight, keeping a log of food ingestion and of physical activity, instruction and encouragement of appropriate diet and physical activity and identification and modification of cues to inappropriate food ingestion and physical activity. There are high rates of attrition and some tendency to weight regain after several months even if the program is continued [545]. However, behavior therapy does moderately enhance weight loss when combined with diet and exercise regimens [546].

Efficacy

Many professionals who work with people seeking to lose weight have an impression that a diversity of conventional treatment programs, various combinations of diet, drugs, exercise and behavior modification, can induce probably significant weight loss in a majority of participants in a few months but frequently there will be some regain of lost weight at one year, more at two years, and by 5 years most of the participants have regained most or all of the weight lost [547]. This trend continues even when the maintenance phase is prolonged. Randomized controlled trials provide some support for this gloomy assessment but there are difficulties and ambiguities in the interpretation of the data [548;549]. A large range of outcomes has been reported. Generally, the more intensive the intervention, the better the reported result and the longer the period of followup, the worse the reported result. When followup is extended to 5 years or longer, most participants do not maintain a weight loss of 5% of initial weight [548]. The diversity of outcomes presumably reflects a large number of factors difficult to evaluate: intensity of intervention, length of followup, the method of recruitment into the study considering baseline weight, ethnicity/race, socioeconomic factors, motive to lose weight, the dropout rate and the rate of loss to followup.

A likely important motivation for dropouts is the marked disparity between dieters' expectations and the achieved weight losses, even in the short term. In one study of women seeking treatment for obesity an expected average of less than 21% of body weight loss was perceived as less than "acceptable" [550]. A sustained loss of 5% to 10% is associated with important health benefits and few dieters will have attained that 5 years after treatment.

Difficulties in establishing efficacy of various programs for bringing about weight loss has not discouraged widespread false and deceptive advertising by manufacturers and distributors of a wide assortment of products promising to bring about rapid, effortless weight loss [551].

From an epidemiologic perspective recent increased efforts to prevent or reverse overweight and obesity have been a definite failure in the United States and perhaps throughout the industrialized world. A survey of 118,000 American adults reported in 1999 [552] that prevalence of attempting to lose or maintain weight was 28.8% and 35.1% among men and 43.6% and 34.4% among women, respectively. Surveys 1988-1994 and 1999-2000 found that in the United States prevalence of obesity (defined by BMI 30 or greater) in adults increased from 22.9% to 30.5%; prevalence of overweight (defined by BMI 25 to 29.9) increased from 55.9% to 64.5% and prevalence of extreme obesity, defined as a BMI greater than 39.9, increased from 2.9% to 4.7% [553]. Using similar methodology in the same population there was no significant decrease in the same categories of adiposity in the intervals represented by 1999-2000 to 2001-2002, following an interval of intense public policy activity by Federal agencies [554]. A publication in 2010 reported a reduction in the United States in the rate of increase of obesity during the last 10 years but no reduction in prevalence [11].

Lack of evidence for efficacy of weight reduction programs prompted the Canadian Task Force on Preventive Health Care to recommend in 1999: "For obese adults without obesity-related diseases, there is insufficient evidence to recommend in favor of or against weight-reduction therapy because of lack of evidence supporting the long-term effectiveness of weight reduction methods…;for obese adults with obesity-related diseases (e.g. diabetes mellitus, hypertension), weight reduction is recommended because it can alleviate symptoms and reduce drug therapy requirements, at least in the short term…" [548]. These guidelines are somewhat more restrictive than those promulgated by the National Institutes of Health in 2000: "Weight loss therapy is recommended for patients with a BMI equal to or greater than 30 and for patients with a BMI between 25 and 29.9 or a high-risk waist circumference and two or more risk factors." [555]. These guide lines are available at www. nhlbi.nih.gov.

The National Weight Control Registry includes more than 4000 self-selected persons who have achieved a documented weight loss of at least 30 lb. (13.6 kg.) and maintained it for at least 1 year. When reported in 2005 they had lost an average of 73 lb. (33 kg.) and maintained a loss of at least 30 lb. (13.6 Kg) for an average of 5.7 years [556]. Principal means employed have been maintained reduced caloric intake, moderate fat intake, frequent monitoring of weight and an exceptional level of physical activity, about 1 hr. daily of moderate-intensity exercise e.g. brisk walking. With the exception of the large exercise component, these devices are mainstays of virtually all conventional treatment, which is much less successful. Consequently it is tempting to conclude that the people in the Registry are different in some important way from the average person undertaking conventional treatment. In a study comparing brain activity as revealed by positron emission activity in successful dieters compared with non-dieters it was concluded: "Cortical areas involved in controlling inappropriate behavioral responses, such as the (dorsal prefrontal cortex), are particularly activated in successful dieters in response to meal consumption. The association between degree of dietary restraint and the coordinated neural changes in the (dorsal prefrontal cortex) and (orbitofrontal cortex) raises the possibility that cognitive control of food intake is achieved by modulating neural circuits controlling food reward." [557]. The origins of these altered neural responses are, of course, unknown. Available data do not permit distinguishing between innate, i.e. genetic, sources and environmentally acquired sources but the fact that these people were previously obese suggests an environmental impact mediating a changed response.

Children

There has been intense interest in the prevention and treatment of overweight and obesity in children. In the assessment interval 1999-2002 16% of American children had a BMI exceeding the 95th percentile value for age and gender [554]. In all the more affluent countries of the world the rates have been rising. Obese children risk becoming obese adults [558], incurring risks of health consequences reviewed in the Chapter MEDICAL HAZARDS OF OBESITY. A significant prevalence of risk factors for cardiovascular disease has been found in obese American children aged 12 to 19 years [559]. Concern has been increased by a statistical forecast that American children, for the first time in history, may not enjoy as many years of life as their parents, as a consequence of obesity and associated morbidities [560].

Obesity in children presents a challenge and a hope. We wish not to impair growth and development with harmful diets and we hope to avoid some of the burden of chronic disease and lethal disease associated with obesity in both children and adults by preventing and treating childhood obesity. Intuitively it seems that we, parents, teachers, the community, could regulate what children eat and regulate their physical activity. Interventions have included recommendations to the food, beverage and restaurant industries, recommendations to food retailers, urging the entertainment and popular media to provide helpful content, attempts to educate parents, teachers, and school authorities and attempts to influence government policy-setting. There have been some limited successes. However, these efforts have not been consistently effective in preventing or remedying overweight and obesity in children even in short intervals [561]. It has been suggested that "chronic care models" are needed, especially for severely obese children [562].

Not surprisingly there has been resistance to change from children, from teachers, from parents, from the school bureaucracy [563] and from the food industry [90]. Major changes are required and cannot be achieved quickly.

The U.S. Preventive Services Task Force has performed an extensive, critical review of the available clinical literature relevant to juvenile obesity. The U.S. Preventive Services Task Force (USPSTF) is an independent panel of non-federal experts in prevention and primary care. In July, 2005 the panel concluded:

"The USPSTF concludes that the evidence is insufficient to recommend for or against routine screening for overweight in children and adolescents as a means to prevent adverse health outcomes....The USPSTF found insufficient evidence for the effectiveness of behavioral counseling or other preventive interventions with overweight children that can be conducted in primary care settings or to which primary care clinicians can make referrals. There is insufficient evidence to ascertain the magnitude of the potential harms of screening or prevention and treatment interventions." [564].

SURGERY

Rising prevalence of obesity in the United States and especially the disproportionate increase in extreme obesity [565] has naturally resulted in an increase in performance of bariatric surgical procedures from 12,775 in 1998 to an estimated greater than 140,000 in 2005 [566]

In February 2006 the Centers for Medicare & Medicaid Services announced that it would pay for certain bariatric surgery procedures as "reasonable and necessary" with certain stipulations. A list of three types of covered operations was given and a list of five not-covered operations was given. The Centers periodically describe itemized coverages as reasonable and medically necessary after extensive review of available literature, evaluation of commissioned studies and reports, and assessments of invited public comments. Policies of the Centers are important because they are likely to be adopted by other third party payers for medical care and tend to set standards of care [567].

Approval is for Medicare beneficiaries who have "a BMI equal to or greater than 35, have at least one comorbidity related to obesity, and have been previously unsuccessful with the medical treatment of obesity". Comorbidities mentioned are hypertension, dyslipidemia, coronary heart disease, stroke, gallbladder disease, osteoarthritis, sleep apnea, respiratory disorders, and endometrial, breast, prostate, and colon cancers.

There has been increasing interest in performance of bariatric surgery in extremely obese adolescents and before irreversible pathologies develop. There are serious ethical problems focusing on informed consent and lack of information about long term outcomes [568].

Efforts to remedy or at least ameliorate obesity by surgery began before 1954. Many of the operations performed earlier are seldom performed in 2006 either because they failed to cause adequate sustained weight loss or because the complications, unintended consequences, were unacceptable. The three types of Medicare-approved operations are Roux-en-Y gastric bypass, laparoscopic adjustable gastric banding, and biliopancreatic diversion with duodenal switch. These operations vary greatly in the anatomical details but all produce large sustained weight losses with amelioration of comorbidities in the candidate populations with what the Medicare authorities have deemed to be acceptable complication rates. Drawings of the anatomical results of the operations have been published [569-571]

Three mechanisms are responsible for the weight loss following the surgeries. Gastric restriction, reducing the capacity of the stomach, produces a sense of satiety after a small meal. Laparoscopic adjustable gastric banding succeeds by gastric restriction. The Roux-en-Y gastric bypass and the biliopancreatic diversion combine gastric restriction and malabsorption. Diversion of the output of the stomach from the normal site, the duodenum, to a lower portion of the digestive tract where nutrients are poorly absorbed causes weight loss by malabsorption. Roux-en-Y surgery, but not gastric banding, results in increased secretion of hormones originating in the small intestine which promote satiety. Experiments in rats confirm that the hormones responsible are peptide YY and glucagon-like peptide-1 [572]. The increase occurs before there has been significant weight loss [573;574] (See the section entitled **Gut Hormones, Satiety Factors** in **CHAPTER 3**).

These three operations all place great demands on the surgeon's skill and experience. Not only are extensive rearrangements of normal anatomy made but the anatomy of obese persons makes obstacles to the surgery. Sometimes specially designed instruments are needed. Postoperative care requires skill, knowledge, and experience from nursing and other institutional personnel. Consequently Medicare requires that the surgery be performed at a facility certified by the American College of Surgeons as a Level 1 Bariatric Surgery Center or at a facility certified by the American Society for Bariatric Surgery as a Bariatric Surgery Center of Excellence. The American College of Surgery and the American Society for Bariatric Surgery have described detailed requirements for certification concerning type of hospital, volume of surgeries performed in the hospital and by the surgeons, surgeon training, education, and credentialing, and facility equipment, and staffing.

Short Term Mortality

Prospective data show that perioperative mortality for patients undergoing gastric bypass is predicted by five variables:

- •BMI equal to or greater than 50,

- •Male gender,

- •High blood pressure,

- •Age greater than 45 years,

- •Risk factors for pulmonary embolism (see **Pulmonary Embolism** in **APPENDIX 2**).

The greater the number of variables present the greater the risk ranging from 0.2% for 0 or 1 to 2.4% for 4 to 5 [575].

Complications specifically related to surgery are leakage of anastomoses, gastrointestinal bleeding, infection, pneumonia, and pulmonary embolism [571].
The increasing progression of risk of mortality is laparoscopic adjustable gastric banding, Roux-en-Y gastric bypass and biliopancreatic diversion. This is also the increasing progression of weight loss .

Long Term Mortality

In comparisons with matched control groups bariatric surgery, generically, reduces mortality for up to 10 years. The improvement is attributable mostly to a reduction in cardiovascular deaths and deaths from cancer.[576-579]. A troubling finding was reported by Adams and colleagues who reported in a study with a 7 year average follow up that the sum of deaths from accidents unrelated to drugs, poisoning of undetermined intent, suicide, and "other" *i.e.* "all nondisease causes", were significantly greater in the gastric bypass group by comparison with a matched control group although total mortality was significantly reduced in the surgical group [580].

Benefits of Surgery

Those who dropout or are otherwise lost to followup have been particularly troublesome. Nearly all programs have been plagued by significant dropout rates, reported to range from 5% to 38% [549]. Investigators have a dilemma when considering how to report their results. If they exclude dropouts from analysis they may tend to make the program seem better than it might otherwise seem to be. Some investigators include dropouts in the final analysis, reporting the initial weight (intention to treat analysis). From a public policy point–of–view this seems plausible but may obscure benefits enjoyed by those who successfully completed the program, although they probably differ significantly from the group as a whole. A third way to report missing data is to use the last value obtained from those who dropped out. This could tend to make the program seem better than it is because dropouts tend to occur early when weight loss is greater than it is at the conclusion of the period of followup. On the other hand perhaps some of those who drop out do so because they have lost little or no weight. Probably the best approach to this problem is for authors to describe their statistical procedures in detail, including an assessment of the error which might result from the methods chosen [581].

This subject is of critical importance for several reasons. There is no doubt that persons with a BMI of 35 or greater, typical surgical candidates, are at risk for obesity-related death [337]. In the industrialized nations the overall prevalence of overweight and obesity has been increasing steadily. In Americans, the most rapid increase is occurring in those persons with BMI of 40 or greater, clinically severe obesity, and a large part of the candidates for bariatric surgery [565]. Similar changes have been occurring in American children [582]. (A man 6 feet (1.82 m) tall who has a BMI of 40 weighs 295 lb (133 kg)). In addition to excess mortality, people this heavy are subject to a long list of distressing experiences. They have a high prevalence of troubling, dangerous comorbidities, diabetes mellitus type II, hypertension, respiratory disorders, and dyslipidemia. Walking is difficult and exhausting. Clothing, chairs, and airline seats do not fit well. Personal hygiene is difficult, unsatisfactory. They have frequent and even chronic skin infections. They experience social and employment discrimination. They feel shame, remorse, and guilt when weight reduction programs fail repeatedly. Dixon and associates found that severely obese subjects are at high risk for depression and that there was sustained reduction of symptoms after weight loss mediated by gastric banding [85].

Obese men have reduced blood concentration of male sex hormone, testosterone, and unsatisfactory libido and sexual performance. Gastric bypass surgery improves hormonal status and quality of sexual life [583].

In a prospective controlled study with average 11 years of followup bariatric surgery reduced the incidence of cancer in obese women but not obese men [584].

Severely obese persons are willing to take some risks to be relieved of at least part of their excess weight. Surgery is the only treatment for obesity which regularly brings about large, sustained weight loss in people with a BMI of 35 or more. The annual rate of performance of bariatric surgery in the United States increased six fold to 14.1 per 100,000 adults from 1990 to 2000. There was little change in in-hospital complication rates [585]. Estimated number of procedures performed in 1990 was 4925 [586] increasing to 72177 in 2002 [587]. Very few of the patients were less than 18 years of age and a somewhat greater number were more than 65 years of age. More than 80% were women [587]. The estimated number of procedures in the United States exceeded 140,000 in 2005 [566].

Weight Loss
It is difficult to make a simple concise statement concerning weight loss following bariatric surgery as a consequence of the heterogeneity of published reports. The amount of weight lost is described as pounds or kilograms lost, as change in BMI, as percentage of patients attaining a BMI of 35, and, most frequently, percentage of excess weight lost. The latter is calculated as (Weight Loss/Excess Weight) times 100 when Excess Weight is (Preoperative Weight less Ideal Weight). Determination of Ideal Weight is not always specified but is presumably from tables of the Metropolitan Insurance Company or the U. S. Department of Agriculture. Presence of comorbidities and outcome of comorbidities are often not described. Sometimes results of different operations are melded. Length of followup has ranged from a few months to 10 years. Length of followup is important because in some studies of longer duration there is a tendency to modest weight regain after the dramatic weight loss of the first year or two. The preoperative weight is very seldom restored [588]. However, people heavy enough to be candidates for bariatric surgery should be aware that when weight stabilizes following surgery, most will still be substantially overweight or frankly obese [589;590].

Meta-analysis of a very large data base with information 1990 to 2006 showed average weight loss 85.5 pounds (38.5 kg) and resolution or improvement of diabetes maintained for 2 years or longer. Rank order of operations was biliopancreatic diversion, gastric bypass and banding [591]. The process of meta-analysis (see **APPENDIX 2**) usually requires substantial selection of the reports analyzed from a much larger group. Consequently these results may not be fully representative of the universe of bariatric surgery. A rigorous comprehensive evaluation of the literature of this subject in 2009 found that surgery produced greater weight loss than conventional treatment and was beneficial for comorbidities but there was only inconclusive evidence concerning outcomes at ten years [592].

Comorbidities

Particular attention has been given to diabetes mellitus, type II, and associated risk factors, hypertension and Dyslipidemia (see **Dyslipidemia** and **Diabetes Mellitus** in **APPENDIX 2**). Most diabetics can expect complete resolution of diabetes II, i.e. normal diagnostic tests and no need for medicines, sometimes within days after surgery, and before significant weight loss has occurred. Most who do not get full resolution can expect improvements. Hypertension and dyslipidemia, often accompanying diabetes mellitus type II, are also frequently resolved or improved. Not surprisingly data regarding outcomes after intervals longer than 10 years are sparse [588;593-595]. Rank order for weight loss and resolution of diabetes is biliopancreatic diversion, Roux-en-Y gastric by pass and banding [596].

Better results are obtained with less severe disease and disease of shorter duration. It is probable that there is a population of diabetics for whom treatment of choice is surgery before irreversible complications occurs. Compared with an equally heavy control group, nondiabetic patients having surgery have a lower incidence of diabetes, dyslipidemia and hypertension [597].

Long Term Complications

Some of the late complications of bariatric surgery are specific for the particular operation performed. Gastric banding may result in slippage of the band from its appropriate site, erosion of the stomach by the band, or infection at the band site. Biliopancreatic diversion presents a high risk of metabolic disorders. Characteristic of Roux-en-Y gastric by pass are stenosis of anastamotic sites resulting in intractable vomiting, pancreatitis, stomach ulcers, loss of bone mass [598] and dumping syndrome (sweating, weakness, mild hypoglycemia, and malaise after eating). For more information, see **Dumping Syndrome** in **APPENDIX 2**: .

A syndrome which shares much with the dumping syndrome has been called hyperinsulinemic neuroglycopenia. It seems most frequently and is best described in subjects who have had Roux-en-Y gastric bypass but has also occurred after other kinds of gastric surgery. The incidence is unknown but is thought to be low. About 1-5 years following gastric bypass the patient, who may or may not have experienced the dumping syndrome, begins having episodes of severe hypoglycemia (low blood glucose) 1-3 hours following a meal. Symptoms have been confusion, loss of consciousness and seizures. The concentration of insulin in blood is elevated, causing low blood glucose (see **Insulin** in **APPENDIX 2**.) The mechanism of this complication has been hypothesized to be accelerated release of factors by cells of the small intestine ("gut hormones") promoting secretion of pancreatic insulin as a consequence of rapid release of gastric contents from the small gastric pouch. Treatments employed have been diet, drugs which inhibit insulin secretion and partial or total pancreatectomy [599-601].

All bariatric operations may result in gall bladder disease, gastroesophageal reflux, incisional hernias, malnutrition, anemia, vitamin deficiency, and calcium deficiency [571]. There is evidence that obesity, preoperatively, is associated with some degree of vitamin D deficiency [602]. Nearly all the late complications of bariatric surgery are potentially manageable, medically or surgically, but require thorough followup, detract from general health and quality of life and add to costs.

Cost Effectiveness

Establishing cost effectiveness is fraught with difficulties. The first is a paucity of appropriate studies. They are difficult to perform. The extent to which publication bias is a factor is unknown. What surgeon wants to publish a study demonstrating that bariatric surgery is *not* cost effective? What costs should be included, *e.g.* time lost from work? What benefits should be included and how should they be weighted, *e.g.* improved quality of life? How long should the time interval be during which the evaluation is made? Presumably some benefits last for life. Should there be a comparison with a no-treatment alternative or with a conventional-treatment alternative?

It seems that in the intermediate term there is not much difference in direct costs between surgically treated and untreated or conventionally treated patients [603-605]. This seems not surprising since the comorbidities of severe obesity are replaced by the morbidities resulting from an expensive, invasive intervention which has severely distorted the gastrointestinal tract. However, when the interval of assessment is extended and benefits are appropriately weighted it appears that a plausible claim of cost effectiveness can be made for bariatric surgery [606-610].

CHAPTER SIX: PUBLIC HEALTH INTERVENTIONS

A growing flood since 1952 of public policy activities has mostly taken the form of attempts to manage the diet and physical activity of children during the hours they are at school, production of reports, guidelines, and educational literature by government agencies, and professional organizations directed toward health care professionals and the general public, mandates for labels on food, demands that the food industry provide quantitatively and qualitatively more healthful food and stop advertising unhealthful food choices, especially those directed toward children, proposals for taxes on soft drinks and snack foods, and proposals for land use and public facilities promoting physical exertion. While there may have been isolated relatively small scale successes, from an epidemiological perspective there is no evidence of an impact on the prevalence of obesity.

Many cities have recently passed laws requiring restaurants information about nutrition, Calorie counts on menus. The public seems to approve.

In 2009 the Centers for Disease Control and Prevention published the findings of an expert panel entitled Recommended Community Strategies and Measurement to Prevent Obesity in the United States. There were 24 evidence-based recommendations. Most required action by governmental entities *e.g.* changes in commercial and residential zoning. Some required significant expenditure of public money e.g. enhancement of infrastructure supporting bicycling [611]. Is there sufficient public demand to effect these changes?

EPILOGUE

Among American adults prevalence of obesity, defined as BMI 30 or greater, increased from 12.8% assessed in the interval 1960-1962 [9] to 32.2% in the interval 2003-2004 [6] and 33.8% in 2007-2008 [11]. Among American children those judged overweight for age and gender increased from 11% in 1988-1994 [612] to 16% in 1999-2002 [554]. Similar trends were present in most age, gender, and race/ethnic groups. A trend to increasing adiposity has occurred in the populations of most nations of the industrialized world.

Unless a safe, effective, passive device, e.g. a drug, is found, the greatest promise for reducing the damaging trend to obesity seems to be in public policy, despite its lack of demonstrated effect. Efforts to reduce the incidence and prevalence of smoking have encountered formidable obstacles, including determined opposition by the wealthy tobacco industry. Nevertheless the prevalence of smoking by American adults has declined from 42.4% in 1965 to 21% in 2004 as a result of a combination of public and private efforts [613]. A similarly prolonged and intense effort may be necessary to combat obesity.

Hill and associates [614] have calculated that the average gain in weight of American adults during the 8 years preceding the year 2000 would have been prevented by consuming 100 Calories per day less. One hundred Calories is substantially less than the caloric value of a can of popular soft drink or one glass of wine. Surely our society can achieve this modest result?

APPENDIX 1

Body Mass Index (weight/height squared, W/H^2) is a mathematical construct associated with many problems. The intention of this device is to accommodate the fact that tall people are expected to weigh more than short people even if not obese, *i.e.* having excess body fat, and short people are expected to weigh less than tall people even if not underweight. The equation for a usually assumed model is:

$W = bH^2$ In which: b = regression coefficient

If the intercept of W on H^2 model is not zero, ratios obtained in this way may result in spurious vales when used to calculate a variety of statistics [53]. It is an observed fact that a non-zero intercept does occur, as it does with most ratios in biomedicine. The equation for the correct model is:

$W = a + bH^2$ In which: a = the value of the intercept on the ordinate.

We may write:

$$\frac{W}{H^2} = \frac{a}{H^2} + b$$

The body mass cannot be calculated by this equation because it contains two unknowns, a and b. This problem and others can be avoided by employment of analysis of covariance. With modern computers the calculations are neither laborious nor difficult but some statistical expertise is required to choose the proper procedure in special situations.

Densitometry is a procedure for the indirect estimation of fat-free component and fat component. The method is also called "underwater weighing" and "hydrodensitometry". It is a measurement of the specific density (weight per unit volume) of the intact human body. Efforts to obtain information about the properties of the human body by measurements of the specific density or gravity of the whole body were begun at least as early as 1814 [615]. Intensive scientific efforts, initiated by American investigators working for the armed forces, began about 1942. Densitometry was among the first indirect methods for studying body composition. It has been frequently used as a criterion method, a "gold standard". Developers of newer methods have attempted to validate them by demonstrating concordance of values obtained with a newer method with values obtained by densitometry.

The fundamental principles of densitometry were discovered by the famous Greek mathematician, scientist, and inventor Archimedes who was born about 285 B.C. and lived and worked in Syracuse in Sicily most of his life. There is a well known and amusing story, regarded by historians as probably apocryphal, about the event of the discovery. The local king, Hieron II, asked Archimedes to measure the amounts of silver and of gold in a metal wreath, non-destructively, of course. While bathing, Archimedes was contemplating the problem when inspiration brought to his mind the basis of a solution. He leaped from his bath and ran nude down the street shouting "Eureka!" ("I have found it!"). To learn more about this fascinating genius visit the Web site; *www.mcs.drexel.edu/~crorres/ Archimedes/contents.html*. (Accessed 03/08/10)

What he found in his well prepared mind was what is now known as Archimedes' principle. A formal statement of it is: an object wholly or partially immersed in a fluid will be buoyed up by a force equal to the weight of the fluid displaced. For present purposes this means that for a human body the difference in weight between a body measured in air and measured while totally immersed in water is equal to the weight of the water displaced. The weight of water is readily converted to a volume by dividing the weight by the known density of water at the temperature at which the procedure is carried out. By definition, the density of that human body is the weight in air divided by the volume of water displaced, which is equal to the volume of the body. In scientific work, units will be kilograms of weight per liter of volume (kg/l).

In research with human subjects, the person to be examined is first weighed in air and is then weighed in a large water-filled tank while completely immersed. Little or no clothing is worn and the volume of air in the lungs, determined by techniques standard in pulmonary medicine, is subtracted from the volume of the body. Thus we have the density of a living, breathing warm human subject.

It is but a step via Archimedes' principle to the idea that if the body being examined consists of two components, the overall gross density will be a consequence of the relative weights of the two components and of their respective densities. In order to make a useful calculation it is necessary to have a numerical value for each of the two densities.

A value of 0.9000 kg/l for the density of the fat component seems generally accepted although the reports providing the information on which that value is based seem to me few in number and sparse in detail. The evidence consists of cadaver analyses and examination of tissues excised at surgery.

Development of a numerical value for the density of the fat-free component has been a difficult challenge. The fat-free component is not an anatomic structure which can be excised and examined. Indeed, it is a multicomponent mathematical abstraction. The value most commonly cited recently is 1.1000 kg/l. The most impressive evidence supporting that value is a synthesis of separate weights and densities of the substances and structures making up the fat-free component obtained from cadaver analysis [616]. Using these values for densities, and some standard algebraic maneuvers it has been possible to develop a mathematical expression for percent body fat for which the only required additional information is the gross density of the human subject. That expression is: % Body Fat = [(4.95/Density) – 4.5] 100, known as Siri's formula after the investigator who first promulgated its application in human studies in 1956. The general approach and basic mathematics had been previously described in animal studies by Morales and collaborators [617] in 1945.

The densitometric approach to the indirect estimation of body fat has an appealing elegance which makes it painful to report that there are serious questions about the validity of the results. Despite the operational complexities, the procedure has been repeatedly shown to be reliable in the statistician's sense of being acceptably reproducible over time in subjects presumed not to have changed. The difficulty is that it is not clear that densitometry accurately measures what it purports to measure: body fat.

In order to have a valid measurement, values of densities assigned to the fat component and to the fat-free component must be accurate and must be the same in all individuals in the population examined. If repeated measurements are made over time, the densities must remain the same over time. Not much concern has been expressed about the density of the fat component. Serious doubt has been expressed about the assumption of a constant density of the fat-free component. It is composed of water, bone and its minerals, other minerals, protein, glycogen and numerous other substances. The most likely way in which constant density might occur seems to be constancy of the relative proportions of water, protein, and minerals, the most abundant constituents of the fat-free body. Otherwise, in order to achieve constant density compensating increases and decreases of higher density and lower density elements must occur. The focus has been on body water and on bone as elements which may be variable from time to time in the same individual and from individual to individual, invalidating the assumption of constant density.

The importance of water was indicated by a small number of cadaver analyses performed before 1953 [618] which showed that water is about 70% of the weight of the body less extracted fat. Clearly there is potential for variation in total body water, all of which is by definition confined to the fat-free component, to have a large effect on the density of the fat-free component and the calculated size of the fat component. Subsequently, every-day observation and many scientific studies have shown that total body water is significantly influenced by age, gender, menstrual status, pregnancy, interval since the last ingestion of water, diet, nutrition, gaining weight, losing weight, degree of adiposity, and numerous diseases of lungs, heart, liver, kidneys, metabolism and blood vessels.

Limited cadaver analysis completed before 1953 suggested that the fat-free component includes, by weight, about 7% bone mineral [619]. This may seem rather a small number but its importance becomes apparent in light of chemical analyses of bone which show that bone mineral has a density of about 3.0 kg/l. Small changes in the amount or density of bone mineral contained within the fat-free component could have significant effects on the density of that component.

More recent studies have shown that skeletal mineral quantity is influenced by age, gender, menopausal status, assorted endocrine disorders, exercise, weight gain, weight loss, degree of adiposity, nutrition, diet, and race.

The Siri formula is very sensitive to the value assigned to the density of the fat-free component. For example, assume that a person has a gross, total body density of 1.050 kg/l, a typical value. The Siri formula as given above, %Body Fat = (4.95/Density - 4.5) 100, would calculate the body fat at 21%, a not unusual value which would not excite suspicion of error. Suppose, however, that the true density of the fat-free component, instead of being the usually assumed value of 1.1000 KG/L, 1.1500 kg/l was used in this calculation. The Siri formula corrected for this value of the density of the Fat-free component, % Body Fat = (4.14/Density - 3.6) 100, yields a calculated value for fat of 34%. If this person weighed 70 kg (155 lb), the first calculation gives 14.7 kg of fat and the second 23.8 kg. The difference, 9.1 kg (20.2 lb), has a stored energy value of about 36,400 Calories. To evaluate the latter consider that a typical daily dietary Caloric intake is about 2000 Calories.

Densitometry requires determination of the gross body density. The calculation is:

$$D = \frac{W_A}{\dfrac{W_A - W_{UW}}{D_W} - RV}$$

in which:

W_A = weight in air

W_{UW} = weight underwater

RV = residual lung volume

D_W = density of water of immersion

Siri's formula is derived by substitution:

$$D_B = \frac{W_A}{V_B} = \frac{(W_F + W_{FF})}{(V_F + V_{FF})} = \frac{(W_F + W_{FF})}{(W_F/D_F + W_{FF}/D_{FF})} = \frac{\dfrac{(W_F + W_{FF})}{W_A}}{\left(\dfrac{W_F/W_A}{D_F} + \dfrac{W_{FF}/W_A}{D_{FF}}\right)}$$

$$D_B = \cfrac{1}{\left(\cfrac{W_F/W_A}{D_F} + \cfrac{W_{FF}/W_A}{D_{FF}}\right)} = \cfrac{1}{\left(\cfrac{W_F/W_A}{D_F} + \cfrac{1-(W_F/W_A)}{D_{FF}}\right)}$$

In which:

V_B = volume of body

W_F = weight of Fat compartment in air

W_{FF} = weight of Fat-free compartment in air

V_F = volume of Fat compartment

V_{FF} = volume of Fat-free compartment

D_F = density of Fat compartment

D_{FF} = density of Fat-free compartment

Taking the reciprocal:

$$\frac{1}{D_B} = \frac{W_F/W_A}{D_F} + \frac{1-\left(W_F/W_A\right)}{D_{FF}}$$

A numerical solution for total body fat (W_F) is possible because all variables in the above equation except W_F have been measured or are have assumed values. W_A and D_B have been measured. D_F and D_{FF} have been assumed to have the values 0.9000 kg/l and 1.1000, respectively.

The difficulties of performing densitometry, the discomfort for the subjects, the time and equipment required, and the uncertain validity of the results has inspired searches for better ways indirectly to estimate body fat.

Doubly Labeled Water provides a means of estimating the rate of production of carbon dioxide, an end product of metabolism of fat, carbohydrate and protein. If the rate of production of carbon dioxide is known and the respiratory quotient, the ratio carbon dioxide produced/oxygen consumed, is measured, or estimated from known properties of the diet, all the equations explicated below for the practice of **indirect calorimetry** are available for probing metabolism. (See below discussion of indirect calorimetry.) The special advantage of doubly labeled water studies is that measurement can be made in free living people over intervals of days or weeks without the restraints of a respiratory chamber or other apparatus of indirect calorimetry.

If deuterium labeled water, heavy water, D_2O, is removed from the body only as water, generically H_2O, the rate of decline of the specific activity of deuterium labeled water, D_2O/H_2O, is an index of the turnover rate of body water. (Turnover rate is the rate at which a constant quantity of a substance is depleted and replenished.) However, isotopic oxygen, ^{18}O, is removed from the body both in water, $H_2{}^{18}O$, and in carbon dioxide, $C^{18}O_2$. Since D is removed only in water and ^{18}O is removed both in water and in carbon dioxide, the difference in turnover rates for D and ^{18}O is the turnover rate for carbon dioxide. The circumstance that ^{18}O is removed from the body both in water and in carbon dioxide is the consequence of isotopic equilibrium of water and carbon dioxide mediated by the enzyme carbonic anhydrase:

$$H_2CO_3 \leftrightarrow H_2O + CO_2$$

In practice known quantities of D_2O and $H_2^{18}O$ are administered orally. At intervals thereafter samples of body water, urine, are collected and the specific activity of D and of ^{18}O are measured by mass spectrometry.

The following exposition of this ingenious model closely follows that of Lifson, Gordon, and McClintock [620;621] who first lucidly presented it in 1955. Their notation is preserved.

$$- dN_D^*/dt = r_{H2O} (N_D^*/N) = r_{H2O} S_D$$

in which:

N_D^* = number of D_2O (heavy water) molecules in the body

N = number of water molecules in the body

r_{H2O} = rate of loss of water molecules from the body

S_D = specific activity of deuterium in body water (N_D^*/N)

t = time

Divide by N:

$$- dS_D/dt = (r_{H2O}/N) S_D = K_D S_D$$

in which:

r_{H2O}/N = fractional deuterium turnover rate in body water, designated K_D

$$- dN_O^*/dt = r_{H2O}(N_O^*/N) + 2r_{CO2} (N_O^*/N) = (r_{H2O} + 2r_{CO2}) S_O$$

In which:

N_O^* = number of water molecules in the body which incorporate isotopic oxygen

$2r_{CO_2}$ = rate of removal of carbon dioxide from the body. The factor 2 is required because each molecule of carbon dioxide includes two atoms of oxygen.

S_O = specific activity of $H_2^{18}O$ in body water

Dividing by N:

$$-dS_O/dt = ((r_{H2O} + 2r_{CO_2}) /N) S_O = K_O S_O$$

in which:

K_O = fractional turnover rate of ^{18}O in body water

$K_O - K_D = (r_{H_2O} + 2r_{O_2})/N - r_{H_2O}/N$

therefore

$K_O - K_D = 2r_{O_2}/N$

$r_{CO_2} = (N/2)(K_O - K_D)$

and

Total $CO_2 = (N/2)(K_O - K_D)\Delta t$

N can be measured by isotope dilution. K_O and K_D are evaluated by the logarithmic decline of specific activity of D and ^{18}O in body water

$-dS/dt = KS$

$-(dS/S)/dt = K = d\ln S/dt$

and

$\Delta\ln S/\Delta t = K$

As in most isotopically based estimates, the use of doubly labeled water to estimate carbon dioxide production requires many assumptions, some of which can be only approximately correct. Perhaps the most important is the steady state assumption, the assumption that over the days, or weeks of the estimate the quantities of water and of carbon dioxide in the body remain constant and their rates of elimination and repletion remain constant. Obviously only a mean value over an adequately long time interval can be a useful approximation. Nevertheless measurement of the rate of production of carbon dioxide for intervals of days or weeks by doubly labeled water compares favorably with simultaneous measurements in the respiratory chamber. The range of uncertainty as a percentage of total production rate has been estimated to be a single digit. Of course, use of the carbon dioxide production rate for estimating energy production and differential substrate oxidation rates according to the concepts of indirect calorimetry requires an additional array of assumptions which are not so easily validated.

Dual Energy Xray Absorptiometry evolved from single photon absorptiometry. Development of single photon absorptiometry for clinical purposes was begun about 1962 as a method of estimating the density of bones in people, especially those with osteoporosis. "Photon" in this context refers not to visible light but to a high-energy, penetrating radiation, a γ-ray (gamma-ray). The usual source of the radiation was americium-241, an element which does not occur in nature but was prepared by the Atomic Energy Commission at the Oak Ridge Laboratory in Tennessee by neutron bombardment of plutonium. The beam radiated by the americium was directed through an arm or a leg and the attenuation of the radiation measured as a quantitative index of the density of the mineral of the bone. A serious difficulty was that the beam was attenuated not only by the bone but also by the surrounding soft tissue. A compensating correction was made by immersing the body part radiated in a relatively large volume of water making uniform, for practical purposes, the non-bone attenuation of the beam. In practice this could work well only in the extremities.

Very soon after the introduction of single photon absorptiometry, dual-photon absorptiometry (DPA) appeared [622] in clinical settings. It had been previously known that in principle the composition of a multicomponent absorber could be estimated by the attenuation of beams at multiple energies. This technology has permitted the simultaneous estimation of fat, bone mineral, and non-fat, non-bone lean body in the intact human body. At first the favored source of radiation was gadolinium-153, a radioactive isotope not found in nature but produced at the Oak Ridge Laboratory. It was soon recognized that use of gadolinium-153 was associated with serious difficulties.

The time period during which the isotope loses one half its radioactivity is 242 days, necessitating yearly replacement. As the source aged, its radioactivity altered in such way that estimates of mass or density of the same substance were altered with time (drifted). The photon beam of Gadolinium-153 has been largely replaced by X-rays produced by electron (cathode ray) bombardment of a metal target in a vacuum tube. The broad spectrum of emitted radiation is narrowed to two major peaks of appropriate energy by filtration with metal, hence the expression Dual Energy X-ray Absorptiometry.

The apparatus consists of a table on which the human subject lies supine with mechanically yoked radiation source below and detectors above, an electromechanical apparatus providing programmable automatic movement of the source-detector assembly, an array of electronic pulse analysis devices and a computer and software for processing of radiation and other data. The source-detector assembly moves to make multiple contiguous transverse scans forming a rectilinear raster composed of pixels of programmable size, similar to a television screen or computer monitor screen. In this way there is made a two dimensional picture of the whole body, made up of thousands of pixels. The differential attenuation of the two energies of radiation for each pixel, separately, provides a basis for calculation of the amount of bone mineral and of soft tissue. Soft tissue can be further resolved into fat and into lean body devoid of bone mineral and fat. The total body amounts of bone, fat, and lean are calculated by adding the amounts of each in all of the pixels. The principles on which these calculations are based are outlined below

A full understanding, in detail, of this very complicated methodology is probably not possible for those of us not educated in radiation physics and radiation technology. However, there are questions which anyone can ask and all interested persons should ask. We can all understand the answer to the general question: "Does it work?" To expand that question we can ask a series of more specific questions which have quantitative answers.

Does the sum of weights of fat, bone mineral and residual lean body, measured by X-ray absorptiometry, equal total body weight measured on a scale? The answer is that there is good correspondence of scale-measured weights and X-ray absorptiometry total weights. Differences occur but usually appear to be small and random. Differences do not seem related to age, gender, or degree of adiposity [36;38;42;623-626]. This corroboration is good news but not definitive. It is possible to obtain concordance of total weights in the presence of systematic compensating errors among the three components, bone, fat, and residual lean body.

Has the accuracy of measurements of the three components been supported by cadaver analysis? This crucial test has not been performed in man and perhaps, for practical reasons, may never be performed. What we have is cadaver analysis of pigs of various sizes after assessment by dual-energy X-ray absorptiometry [21;23-29;627]. Pigs were chosen because they are readily available in sizes comparable to humans of all ages; because their body composition, fat, water, bone, is similar to that of humans; and because in a very general way their morphology is of the same category as that of humans, four extremities, and a central mass. Other resemblances which might be thought to exist are not relevant to this discussion.

Briefly, in general and without respect to species, x-ray absorptiometry is reliable in the statisticians' sense that, when thorough quality assurance measures are established and diligently pursued, repeated measurements of the same unchanging subject over intervals of months [628] or years [629] are acceptably similar. X-ray absorptiometry is precise in the common meaning that measurements of a subject before and after an intervention producing a small known change can be shown by x-ray absorptiometry to be appropriately different. The variations observed in serial replicate measurements of body components in the same individual are a small fraction of the average values. On that basis one would expect and it has been shown that small changes in body composition in people, brought about by dieting [629;630] or intravenous infusion of water or withholding of water [629;631] or hemodialysis [632;633] result in clear changes in x-ray-derived values. Reliability and precision are desirable characteristics of any measuring system. That is the good news about X-ray absorptiometry. The bad news is most clearly demonstrated in the studies of pigs. It has to do with a property of measurements which in ordinary language is called validity or accuracy. A valid measurement is one which measures what it purports to measure, within acceptable limits.

In the pig studies results obtained by X-ray scanning have been compared with results obtained by direct physical and chemical analysis of the carcasses of pigs of weights ranging from that of premature human infants to that of adult humans. It is very difficult briefly to summarize these data. The hardware and software used in dual energy absorptiometry have been subjected to continuous engineering development for 30 years and, doubtless, is ongoing. The studies of pigs, of which there have been at least 10, have been performed with different systems from the same and different manufacturers [21;23-27;29;634-636]. Different presentations of data and different statistical treatments cause problems in making comparisons.

Generalizing, it can be said that estimates of total body mass, the sum of bone, fat, and lean body, compared well with weights obtained by scale, were precise, and accurate. Measurement of total body bone mineral had poor accuracy in the smallest animals and was improved in the larger animals. Virtually all studies showed significant underestimation or overestimation of fat in comparison with chemical values, often with poor precision.

The conclusion, which some researchers have drawn, based on these and other findings, that dual energy x-ray absorptiometry has serious deficiencies, making its use questionable for study of fat, is based on the assumption that the results of measurements in pigs reflect those obtained in humans [28;627]. This assumption may be incorrect. However, alternative means of validating x-ray absorptiometry measurements are not attractive. There are numerous studies comparing results obtained with x-rays with values obtained by other indirect methods of assessing human body composition, hydrodensitometry, total body potassium, total body water, bioelectric impedance and others. There has been little agreement [31]. The results of these studies are of interest to researchers but the stubborn fact remains that a method of doubtful accuracy cannot be validated by comparing the results with those obtained by other methods known or suspected to lack validity.

Machines and software for dual energy x-ray absorptiometry are widely distributed because they have become the method of choice for estimating bone mineral density and total body bone mineral content, measures of central importance in assessing the common disorder osteoporosis and its treatment. For this purpose some deficiencies are known which need not be discussed in this document which is about fat. The scans are completed in less than one-half hour and the dose of radiation is less than that received as cosmic radiation during a five hour flight in a commercial airliner [28;637]. Perhaps there will be improvements in the software and hardware and the uncertainties about the circumstances in which accurate or inaccurate measurements are to be expected will be dissipated by more and better data.

Dual Energy X-ray Absorptiometry has its scientific basis in Lambert's law of absorption which is: For a monoenergetic source of radiation traversing a homogeneous absorber, each layer of equal thickness absorbs an equal fraction of the radiation traversing it.

The mathematical expression of this relationship is:

$$I = I_0 e^{-ux}$$

or

$$\ln(I_0/I) = ux$$

in which:

I = intensity of the attenuated X-ray beam.

I_0 = intensity of the unattenuated, incident, x-ray beam

u = mass absorbance coefficient (cm²/gm)

x = mass per unit area (gm/cm²)

For a binary absorber having components a and b:

$$\ln(I_0/I) = u_a M_a + u_b M_b$$

in which:

u_a = absorption coefficient for component a

M_a = mass of component a

u_b = absorption coefficient for component b

M_b = mass of component b

Given radiation of two intensities, for example:

38 keV, I_0^{38} and 70 keV, I_0^{70}

We may write:

$$\ln\left(I_0^{38}/I^{38}\right) = u^{38}_a M_a + u^{38}_b M_b$$

and

$$\ln\left(I_0^{70}/I^{70}\right) = u^{70}_a M_a + u^{70}_b M_b$$

For practical application in estimating differentially the mass of bone and the mass of soft tissue:

$a = B$ = the nonvolatile residuum of bone after prolonged heating at temperature exceeding 500 ^0C.

And

$b = S$ = soft tissue

Solve the above immediately preceding logarithmic equations simultaneously to obtain: "

$$M_S = \frac{u_B^{38} \ln\left(I_0^{70}/I^{70}\right) - u_B^{70} \ln\left(I_0^{38}/I^{38}\right)}{u_B^{38} u_S^{70} - u_B^{70} u_S^{38}}$$

and

$$M_B = \frac{u_S^{70} \ln\left(I_0^{38}/I^{38}\right) - u_S^{38} \ln\left(I_0^{70}/I^{70}\right)}{u_B^{38} u_S^{70} - u_S^{38} u_B^{70}}$$

These equations cannot be solved in this form because the absorption coefficients for soft tissue, u_S, vary from pixel to pixel depending on the relative amounts of fat and lean substance in the pixel (see below.).

Let:

$$R_B = \frac{\mu_B^{38}}{\mu_B^{70}} = \frac{\ln\left(I_0^{38}/I^{38}\right)}{\ln\left(I_0^{70}/I^{70}\right)} \qquad \text{for bone mineral ash only,}$$

and

$$R_S = \frac{\mu_S^{38}}{\mu_S^{70}} = \frac{\ln\left(I_0^{38}/I^{38}\right)}{\ln\left(I_0^{70}/I^{70}\right)} \qquad \text{for pixels from which bone is absent.}$$

We may now write:

$$M_S = \frac{R_B \ln\left(I_0^{70}/I^{70}\right) - \ln\left(I_0^{38}/I^{38}\right)}{R_B \mu_S^{70} - \mu_S^{38}}$$

and

$$M_B = \frac{\ln\left(I_0^{38}/I^{38}\right) - R_S \ln\left(I_0^{70}/I^{70}\right)}{\mu_B^{38} - R_S \mu_B^{70}}$$

R_B and u_B values are invariant in these equations because bone mineral ash is largely the chemically defined substance calcium hydroxyapatite. Their values can be obtained from measurements in phantoms, a more or less anthropomorphic contrivance used to test, measure, or calibrate radiological machines. However, in order to calculate it is necessary also to have values for the absorption coefficients and the ratio of absorption coefficients for soft tissue. Weighted mean values for $\overline{R}_S$, $\overline{\mu}_S^{38}$, and $\overline{\mu}_S^{70}$ are computed for all pixels in which bone is absent. These values are used to compute, for each pixel, M_S and M_B. The sum of the values is the total body bone mineral ash and total body soft tissue.

Soft tissue can be divided into lean and fat components as a consequence of the linear relation of fractional lean content (and fractional fat content) with R_S.

We may write:

$$R_S = \frac{\mu_f^{38} M_f + \mu_l^{38} M_l}{\mu_f^{70} M_f + \mu_f^{70} M_l}$$

In which:

u_f^{38} = absorption coefficient at 38 keV for fat only
u_l^{38} = absorption coefficient at 38 keV for lean only
u_f^{70} = absorption coefficient at 70 keV for fat only
u_l^{70} = absorption coefficient at 70 keV for lean only
M_f = mass of fat
M_l = mass of lean
keV = thousand electron Volts

Values for absorption coefficients can be determined in phantoms.

Let:

$$F = \frac{M_f}{M_f + M_l}$$

$$L = \frac{M_l}{M_f + M_l} = 1 - F$$

Consequently:

$$R_S = \frac{\mu_f^{38} F + \mu_l^{38} L}{\mu_f^{70} F + \mu_l^{70} L}$$

It is an empirical fact that: $u_f^{70} \cong u_l^{70}$

Let:

μ_{fl}^{70} = the combined μ^{70}

$$R_f = \frac{\mu_f^{38}}{\mu_{fl}^{70}}$$

$$R_l = \frac{\mu_l^{38}}{\mu_{fl}^{70}}$$

We may now write:

$$R_S = \frac{\mu_f^{38} F + \mu_l^{38} L}{\mu_{fl}^{70}}$$

and

$$R_S = R_f F + R_{fl}(1 - F)$$

$$F = \frac{\overline{R}_S - R_l}{R_f - R_l}$$

From these relations total body fat, total body lean, total body soft tissue and total body bone mineral ash can be computed as fractions of total body weight, or as kilograms. Similar calculations can be made for delineated regions of the body.

The scientific principles underlying dual energy absorptiometry, of which the above is a simplified and truncated exposition, are generally accepted. Complicating the application of these principles is a host of difficult problems of an engineering or technical nature. Examples are instrument drift, counting errors, computational options, misalignment of pixels, motion of the subject, too small scanning tables, composition and maintenance of calibration devices and phantoms, beam morphology, and "beam hardening" (preferential attenuation of lower energy components of polyenergetic x-rays). Additional difficulties are found in the fact that there are three manufacturers of dual energy x-ray systems, each providing proprietary hardware and soft ware. Limited available data consistently show significant differences between values obtained with products from different manufacturers [633;638-640;640;641;641] It is customary to recommend that values obtained with one system be compared only with values obtained with the same system.

Fat Cell Number was estimated by Hirsch and Gallian [642] in samples of adipose tissue obtained from subcutaneous sites by needle aspiration with local anesthesia and in surgical biopsies taken at intraabdominal sites during necessary surgery. The specimen was divided into two parts and each was weighed. The fat content of one part was determined by conventional chemical means. The other part was treated with osmium tetroxide which caused the fat cells to separate from the matrix of connective tissue, nerves and blood vessels which are present in adipose tissue. The separated fat cells were suspended in liquid and counted in a standard commercially available machine used for routine counting of blood cells. In this way the total number of fat cells in a weighed quantity of adipose tissue was determined. Measurement of the total quantity of fat by chemical means in the other weighed sample allowed calculation of the fractional fat content of the adipose tissue at that site. The average fat per cell could then be calculated.

$$\frac{Fat}{Cell} = \frac{SampleWeight \times FractionalLipid}{SampleCells}$$

In the above equation the sample referred to is the osmium tetroxide treated sample. In a subject whose total body fat had been estimated by whatever means, division of total body fat by fat per cell gives an estimate of the total number of fat cells in the body.

Four Component Model is an example of an approach to indirect estimate of body composition which has been called the multicomponent model. In this model independent measurements of separate components are made by combinations of the above methods and the results are mathematically integrated to yield a value for total body fat or some other desired value. A four component model is based on estimate of the fat component and the fat-free component by measurement of body density as described above, total body water by isotope dilution, and total body bone ash by dual energy X-ray absorptiometry [30-32]. The assumptions of constancy of the fat-free component are avoided but other assumptions are required for the calculations.

Those assumptions are:

- In all people at all times total body weight is sufficiently accurately represented by the sum of total body fat, total body protein, total body water, and total body mineral.

- In all people at all times the average density of total body fat is 0.9007 kg/l.

- In all people at all times the average density of total body protein is 1.340 kg/l.

- In all people at all times the average total body bone mineral is 104% of the total body bone ash which is the substance measured by dual energy x-ray absorptiometry and is the non-volatile residuum obtained by prolonged heating of bone at 500 °C.

• In all people at all times the average total body non-osseous mineral is 23.5% of the total body bone ash.

• In all people at all times the average density of total body bone mineral is 2.982 kg/l.

• In all people at all times the average density of total body non-osseous mineral is 3.317 kg/l

The assumption that total body weight is the sum of total fat, total protein, total water and total bone mineral is known to be inaccurate since it does not include glycogen and other carbohydrates. The error may not be large and may not be significant, depending on the use which is made of the estimates of body components. The assumption that total body fat has a density of 0.9007 kg/l rests on measurements of surgical specimens in humans and a variety of laboratory and domestic animals. The consensus is that it is a good value for adipose tissue but inaccurate for the fats of muscle and nervous system. The inaccuracy may be of little significance in well-nourished people in whose bodies most of the fat is present in the adipose tissues under the skin and around the viscera [643-645]. The value 1.340 kg/l for the density of total body protein has been repeatedly cited in the literature. I have not been able to find empirical justification for that number. The earliest mention of it which I have found is in a 1956 paper by the pioneer student of human body composition W. E. Siri who wrote "Proteins vary in density, and the value of 1.340 gm/cc is an average for fully hydrated protein in vitro. Whether or not it is the correct average for human protein in vivo has not been demonstrated." [646]. The assumption that total body bone mineral is 104% of total body bone ash and the density of that ash is 2.982 kg/l rests upon measurements of cow and dog bones [645]. Assumptions that average total body non-osseous mineral is 23.5% of total body bone ash and that the average density of the total body non-osseous mineral rest upon complex calculations in which multiple assumptions are made using data from chemical analyses of four cadavers.

A four-component model, described by Heymsfield and collaborators [32] for indirect estimation of body fat requires measurement of total body density as described above in the section explaining Densitometry, total body bone ash by dual energy X-ray absorptiometry as described above in the section explaining **Dual X-ray absorptiometry**, and total body water by isotope dilution as described below in the section explaining **Isotope Dilution**.

Assume that body weight is the sum of four components:

$$BW = F + P + A + M$$

in which:

BW = body weight
F = weight of total body fat
P = weight of total body protein
A = weight of total body water
M = weight of total body mineral

From the Archimedean principle:

$$\frac{1}{D} = \frac{f}{d_f} + \frac{p}{d_p} + \frac{a}{d_a} + \frac{m}{d_m}$$

in which:

D = total body density
f = fraction of total body weight which is fat

d_f = density of total body fat

p = fraction of total body weight which is protein

d_p = density of total body protein

a = fraction of total body weight which is water

d_a = density of water

m = fraction of total body weight which is mineral

d_m = density of total body mineral

Let: $p = 1 - f - a - m$

Substituting: $\dfrac{1}{D} = \dfrac{f}{d_f} + \dfrac{1}{d_p} - \dfrac{f}{d_p} - \dfrac{a}{d_p} - \dfrac{m}{d_p} + \dfrac{a}{d_a} + \dfrac{m}{d_m}$

D and a are measured quantities.

Assume:

$d_f = 0.9007$ kg/l

$d_p = 1.340$ kg/l

$d_a = 0.9937$ kg/l

A numerical solution for f in the above equation is not possible because m and d_m are unknown. However, dual energy X-ray absorptiometry can measure total body bone mineral ash, the substance produced when bone is heated, resulting in loss of labile substances.

Given:

$M = M_b + M_{no}$

in which:

M_b = weight of total bone mineral before heating

M_{no} = weight of total nonosseous mineral

Assume:

$M_b = 1.0436 TBBA$

$M_{no} = 0.235 TBBA$

in which:

$TBBA$ = weight of total body bone mineral ash

$M = 1.0436 TBBA + 0.235 TBBA = 1.279 TBBA$

Given:

$d_m = \dfrac{M}{MV} = \dfrac{M_b + M_{no}}{MV}$

in which:

MV = volume of M

$$MV = \frac{M_b}{d_{m_b}} + \frac{M_{no}}{d_{m_{no}}}$$

Consequently:

$$d_m = \frac{1.279TBBA}{\dfrac{M_b}{d_{m_b}} + \dfrac{M_{no}}{d_{m_{no}}}}$$

Assume:

d_{m_b} = 2.982 kg / l

$d_{m_{no}}$ = 3.317 kg / l

$$d_m = \frac{1.279TBBA}{\dfrac{1.0436TBBA}{2.982} + \dfrac{0.235TBBA}{3.317}}$$

$$m = \frac{M}{BW}$$

The equation:

$$\frac{1}{D} = \frac{f}{d_f} + \frac{1}{d_f} - \frac{f}{d_p} - \frac{a}{d_p} - \frac{m}{d_p} + \frac{a}{d_a} + \frac{m}{d_m}$$

can thusly have a numerical solution for f.

Impedance is that property of a conductor of electricity which impairs the spread of alternating current in a conductor. When the conductor is material of biologic origin, e. g. a human body, it has been called "bioelectrical impedance." Although even in simple physical systems impedance is a complex phenomenon, machines are available which can measure it, conveniently. Analysis of bioelectrical impedance has been used for study of human body composition. In practice, electrodes are applied, usually to wrists and ankles, and an imperceptible, harmless, alternating current of known frequency and amperage is applied, briefly. While the current flows a meter displays impedance values. In an electrical circuit of simple geometry, some of the factors which influence the observed values are: the length of the conductor, cross sectional area of the conductor, specific resistivity (ohms/centimeter), the frequency of the current, the presence of both parallel and series elements, and inductance and capacitance of the circuit. The human body, viewed as an electrical circuit, presents daunting analytical difficulties as a consequence of its complicated geometry and the varied elements of which it is composed.

It is easy intuitively to imagine that impedance could be an index of some property of body water since the body water is a salt solution and a good conductor of electricity. If the amount of total body water could be estimated from the value for impedance, and if it is assumed that water is a constant fraction of the fat-free component, in the population in which measurements are made, between individuals, and from time to time, one can calculate the fat-free component as the product of some constant and the quantity of total body water. The fat component is, of course, the difference between body weight and the fat-free component.

Isotope dilution is the criterion method for estimation of total body water (see **Isotope Dilution** below for details.) An isotope of an atom is a different atom of similar chemical properties and electron composition to the first, but having an altered nucleus resulting in a different atomic weight. For example, two common hydrogen atoms, together with one atom of oxygen, form the ordinary water molecule (H_2O). These hydrogen atoms have one electron, and a nucleus containing one proton, with an atomic weight of approximately 1. A different isotope of hydrogen, named deuterium, has one electron, and a nucleus containing one proton and one neutron. It has an atomic weight of approximately 2. Water in which deuterium has been substituted for hydrogen, heavy water, D_2O, has been used for estimation of total body water. A known volume of ordinary water containing a known concentration of heavy water is administered to the experimental subject orally or intravenously. Several hours later, after the heavy water has mixed and equilibrated with the body water of the subject, a sample of the subject's body water, as blood, saliva or breath condensate, is obtained. The extent to which the ratio of deuterium to hydrogen in the subject's body water is reduced by comparison with the ratio in the ingested or injected volume of water, the extent of dilution, is a measure of total body water. The mass of total body water can be calculated by simple arithmetic. Measurements of the concentrations of heavy water are made with a complicated and expensive machine and require care, training, and skill. Accuracy of measurement of total body water by isotope dilution has been directly confirmed by desiccation studies of whole bodies in animals. A frequently used variant of this procedure is use of tritiated water, water in which hydrogen of water is substituted by tritium, a radioactive isotope of hydrogen which can be easily measured by its radioactivity.

Attempts have been made to measure total body water by analysis of bioelectrical impedance. A variety of studies are available in which estimates of total body water by bioelectrical impedance analysis have been compared with simultaneous measurements by isotope dilution [647-652]. Most authors have been pleased with the correspondence of values obtained by impedance measurements with values obtained by isotope dilution. Other authors were not gratified. Piccoli and associates [653] have reported evidence that in persons with fluid overload bioelectric impedance analysis generates "absurd values". Experimental conditions and techniques have varied and kinds of populations studied have been different. It is beyond the scope of this document to offer a detailed, technical critique of this subject. I discuss it at this length only because a belief that bioelectrical impedance is a reasonably accurate index of total body water has been central to thinking about the attempted use of impedance measurements for estimation of the fat-free component and, therefore, of the fat component. There is reason to doubt that the belief is always correct.

If the fraction of the fat-free component which is water were known, and if the total body water were known, the fat-free component could be calculated as total body water divided by the fraction of fat-free component which is water. A value of 0.73 has been cited as an approximation of the fractional water content of the fat-free body. This number is derived largely from studies of laboratory animals [654] and a small number of direct chemical analyses of whole human bodies. The uncertainty of the value in man, and the belief, fully justified, that it varies widely in physiological and pathological states has discouraged use of this means of estimating fat-free and fat components.

Serious efforts to estimate the two components using bioelectrical impedance analysis without reference to total body water, were first described in 1985 [655;656]. Principal focus has been on using densitometry as the criterion method. The goal has been to manage impedance analysis so that it "predicts" the results obtained by densitometry performed in the same subjects at the same time. Emphasis has been on the calculations performed to get values for the fat component mass and the fat-free component mass from impedance data rather than on the mechanics of performance of the procedure. Obtaining a value for impedance seems simple. Two electrodes are attached to a wrist and two electrodes are attached to the ankle on the same side of a supine subject. The current is turned on and the impedance value read from a dial. However, various investigators have shown that values obtained for impedance are significantly influenced by the type of electrode, placement of electrodes, body position, ambient temperature, recent physical activity, and the electrical properties of the table on which the subject is lying. Nevertheless, some investigators have demonstrated that it is possible to obtain consistent impedance values with repeated measurement of the same subjects on the same day or with serial measurement of the same subjects on successive days. Several machines from different manufacturers have been available in Europe and the United States. There has been little assessment of differences in results obtained by machines from different manufacturers or different models from the same manufacturer.

However, the principal difficulties in the use of bioelectrical impedance analysis for estimation of body composition have not been thought to reside in the operational details of measurement of impedance. The problem is more fundamental. Few investigators have found that impedance values, alone or corrected for height, can satisfactorily predict fat-free component estimated by densitometry. Impedance apparently does not contain enough information or sufficiently accurate information to predict the densitometric fat-free component. Additional information, additional variables, additional measurements, have been introduced into the calculations by stepwise **Multiple Regression Analysis** (see below in **APPENDIX 1**). This is a statistical method used to construct predictive equations by stepwise inclusion of additional measurements, i. e. variables. For example, it is possible to write an equation for prediction of the densitometric fat- free component which includes in addition to impedance, age, and/or height, and/or body weight. Any characteristic of the subject which can be expressed as a number or to which a number can be assigned can be included. A binary characteristic, gender, can be included by coding, male = 0, female = 1. Some of the variables used by various authors to improve Predictive Equations include, in addition to impedance: gender, age, height, weight, circumferences measured in extremities and trunk, and sums of various **Skin Fold Thicknesses** (see below).

Stepwise multiple regression analysis not only permits inclusion of additional variables in calculation but also permits assessment of the relative importance of each variable included. It is reasonable to ask if inclusion of a term for impedance is justified when numerous other variables are required to obtain an acceptable result. At least four groups of investigators have expressed doubt [657-660].

However, for me, the most damning criticism of impedance-analysis-based estimates of body composition has been the failure to demonstrate credible assessments of changes in body composition brought about by fasting or low caloric diets[630;660-664].

Perhaps the best way to provide a final summary of this perhaps too long and too detailed treatment of bioelectric impedance analysis of body composition is briefly to review the National Institutes of Health Technology Assessment Conference Statement of December 12-14, 1994 entitled *Bioelectrical Impedance Analysis in Body Composition Measurement*.[665]. Little has changed with regard to this technology since 1994 except a reduction in the rate of publication and, I think, an increase in skepticism about the results.

From time to time the National Institutes of Health convenes a panel of experts concerning a particular technology. The panel invites presentations by prominent active investigators using and studying the technology of interest. The panel then develops a consensus and issues a technology assessment statement. Conclusions reached by the panel included:

1. "Precisely what bioelectric impedance analysis measures in terms of electrical and biological parameters is not known and probably varies somewhat from person to person."

2. "Discussions of bioelectrical impedance analysis reports often include a discussion of 'equations'. These equations are those describing the statistical relationships found for a particular population and are not derived from biophysical reasoning…The consequence is that each equation is useful only for subjects that are a close match to the reference population used in the original derivation of the equation."

3. "The panel neither heard nor identified any particular reason why the bioelectrical impedance analysis measurement is other than safe... It does seem wise to advise anyone with an Implanted defibrillator to avoid bioelectrical impedance analysis evaluation..." (see **APPENDIX 2**)

4. "The geometric proportions of obese individuals compared with leaner individuals are such that a greater proportion of body mass and body water is accounted for by the trunk in relation to the extremities; the trunk, however, contributes a relatively minor amount to total body impedance. This situation would tend to result in overestimation of body fat from standard equations."

5. "Available information indicates that bioelectrical impedance analysis is not useful in measuring acute changes in body fat in individuals, although it can characterize longer term changes in groups of subjects".

6. "Bioelectrical impedance analysis provides a reliable estimate of total body water under most conditions. Subsequent estimation of Fat-free Mass and the percentage of body fat vary in validity depending on the population or individual studied and the applicability of the predictive equation used to estimate these parameters of body composition. Bioelectrical impedance analysis can be a useful technique for body composition analysis in healthy individuals and in those with a number of chronic conditions such as mild-to-moderate obesity, diabetes mellitus type II, and other medical conditions in which major disturbances of water distribution are not prominent." (see **Diabetes Mellitus** in **APPENDIX 2**).

My requests for validating data to manufacturers of bioelectrical impedance analyzers for home use elicited no response [666;667]. I suspect that use of such devices provides no information more valuable than that which can be obtained by stepping on the bathroom scale.

Bioelectrical Impedance is best understood by examining the equations which describe its quantitative relationships.

The fundamental expression for series circuits is:

$$Z = \rho \frac{L}{A}$$

in which:

$Z =$ impedance (Ω)

$\rho =$ specific conductivity $\left(\dfrac{\Omega}{cm}\right)$

$L =$ length of conductor (cm)

$A =$ cross sectional area of conductor (cm^2)

Multiplying by $\left(\dfrac{L}{L}\right)$ gives: $\quad Z = \rho \dfrac{L^2}{AL}$

AL is the volume, $V(cm^3)$, of a cylindrical conductor.

Rearranging:

$$V = \rho \frac{L^2}{Z}$$

When the human body is the conductor, $H^2 \left(cm^2 \right)$ height squared, is used as a surrogate for L^2. Not only do the dimensions of the conductor and the specific conductivity influence the impedance but also, in a complex medium like the human body, the capacitance. The fundamental equation is:

$$Z = \sqrt{R^2 + X_c^2}$$

in which:

R = resistance (Ω)

X_c = capacitative reactance (Ω)

At high current frequencies X_c becomes relatively small and is omitted from calculations by some investigators. For the benefit of the engineers among us: R is the sum of the in-phase vectors and X_c is the sum of out-of-phase vectors.

Indirect Calorimetry requires measurement of the rates of oxygen consumption and carbon dioxide production. To accomplish this, the subjects head is enclosed in a hood, sealed to the skin of the neck, into which ambient air, consisting of 21% oxygen and 79% nitrogen, is pumped. For studies of longer duration the whole body of the subject may be enclosed in a small chamber. The gases within the hood or chamber are pumped out through a system of sensors which monitor volume flow, carbon dioxide concentration and oxygen concentration. From these data the rate of oxygen uptake and rate of carbon dioxide production can be calculated. Studies of biochemical intermediates combined with thermodynamic investigations have yielded parameters used in calculation of amounts of substrate oxidized and amounts of energy produced. The principal data are shown in the table below:

Typical Substrate	Oxygen consumed l/gm	Carbon dioxide produced l/gm	Respiratory quotient RQ	Calories/gm oxidized
Carbohydrate	0.746	0.746	1.00	3.74
Fat	2.0191	1.427	0.70	9.46
Protein	0.966	0.774	0.80	4.32

We may write:

$$V_{O_2} = 0.746C + 2.02F + 0.966P$$

$$V_{CO_2} = 0.746C + 1.43F + 0.774P$$

$$N = 0.16P$$

In which:

V_{O2} = rate of oxygen consumption (l/min)
V_{CO2} = rate of oxygen consumption (l/min)
C = rate of oxidation of carbohydrate (gm/min)
F = rate of oxidation of fat (gm/min)
P = rate of oxidation of protein (gm/min)
N = rate of urinary excretion of nitrogen (gm/min)

It is assumed that protein is 16% by weight nitrogen and that the appearance of a nitrogenous substance in the urine is the consequence of oxidation of the corresponding amount of protein.

Simultaneous solution of the above two equations allows us to write:

$$C = 4.57 V_{O2} - 3.23\ V_{O2} - 2.60\ N$$
$$F = 1.69\ V_{O2} - 1.69\ V_{CO2} - 2.03\ N$$
$$P = 6.25\ N$$

Summing the products of the oxidation rates of the three substrates, carbohydrate, fat, and protein, and their respective caloric equivalents gives the rate of energy expenditure.

Rate of energy expenditure $= 3.74\ C + 9.46\ F + 4.32\ P$

If the caloric equivalents of the mixture of substances ingested as food or the caloric equivalents of the mixture of substrates oxidized varies significantly from those employed in the calculations, large errors are possible. These and other sources of error have been evaluated by Livesey and Elia [668] who judged that 5% is the minimum error to be expected of energy estimates by indirect calorimetry.

Isotope Dilution is a valid measure of the volume of a space only if the isotope-bearing substance, the "labeled" substance, is uniformly distributed through the space. If a chemical reaction or an exchange process occurs such that a part of the label is not distributed uniformly, the apparent volume measured, the virtual space will be erroneous. Theoretical considerations and some desiccation data indicate that this is the case for deuterium-labeled water. The error has been estimated to be less than 5% of the measured volume and is attributed largely to exchange reactions of the deuterium with hydrogen in protein [669]. The generic equation for dilution measurements is:

$$V_f = \frac{C_i Vi}{C_f}$$

in which:

V_f = the final volume, the virtual volume estimated by dilution
V_i = the initial volume of labeled substance administered
C_i = the concentration of label in the substance administered
C_f = the concentration of label after dilution in the virtual volume

A correction must be made to account for the amount of isotope excreted in urine during the interval of equilibration. This done by subtracting the amount in the urine from the amount administered, the numerator in the above equation.

Calculation of an estimated Fat-free component assuming a constant value for the fraction of Fat-free component which is water and using a measured volume of total body water, no matter how measured can be accomplished by:

$$TBW = 0.732\,FFM$$

rearranging:

$$FFM = \frac{TBW}{0.732}$$

in which:

FFM = Fat-free component
TBW = total body water

Multiple Regression Analysis has a complexity which forbids communication of only the flavor by a short list of equations or sentences. Fortunately, a slender volume written by Sam Kash Kachigan provides helpful understanding for persons with no more preparation in mathematics than a dimly recalled course of algebra [670].

Neutron Activation Analysis was developed after two nuclear reactor accidents in August, 1945 and May, 1946 at the Los Alamos Scientific Laboratory in which a total of 10 persons were subjected to intense bursts of neutrons and gamma rays. Two people died and others experienced various degrees of radiation injury. These accidents and their victims were studied intensively. Serious efforts were made to estimate the neutron dose received by each person.

When the natural isotope of sodium (^{23}Na), is subjected to neutron bombardment some of it is converted to ^{24}Na in a dose dependent manner. ^{24}Na is a radioactive element which emits gamma rays (X-rays) of a characteristic energy. Measurement of those gamma rays can be used to measure the amount of ^{24}Na present. ^{24}Na was found in the blood and urine of people accidentally irradiated in the Los Alamos accidents [671]. Similarly, ^{24}Na was demonstrated to be present in the urine, blood and whole bodies of persons radiated in a reactor accident at the Hanford Laboratories in 1963 [672].

If, in response to neutron bombardment, the extent of conversion of ^{23}Na to ^{24}Na is a measure of a dose of neutrons, it must be the case that in response to a known dose of neutrons, the amount of ^{24}Na formed is an index of the amount of ^{23}Na irradiated. This principle was the basis of the report by Anderson and collaborators of the first *in vivo* neutron activation analysis of human body composition in 1964 [673].

Presciently, the authors enunciated a problem which has been the stimulus for much of the engineering development of this technique ever since: "What is required is an equal probability that any atom of sodium in the body will be activated and detected—*i.e.*, the product of probability of activation and probability of detection (counting efficiency) shall be substantially the same for all such atoms." Achievement of this goal must somehow overcome the obstacles of irregular geometry of the human body presenting varying thicknesses of different tissues which attenuate the penetration of neutrons and impede the detection of the induced gamma rays. Solutions have been ingenious, elaborate, expensive, and apparently effective. Examples have been neutron radiation in front and in back, or one side and then the other, and positioning of detectors of differing efficiency over parts of the body differing in attenuation of gamma rays.

The principles first applied to measurement of total body sodium have now been extended to measurement in humans of total body carbon, nitrogen, calcium, phosphorous, and chlorine. Atoms excited by neutron bombardments emit gamma rays and undergo one or more nuclear transformations in decay to a stable state.

Validation of measurements by neutron activation analysis has been performed by cadaver analysis in only two human bodies. Knight, in New Zealand, reported results of measurements of nitrogen and of chloride by neutron activation in two cadavers followed by chemical assay [674]. Agreement was excellent. Extensive work estimating accuracy has been performed in phantoms with encouraging results. (A phantom, for radiologists, is an anthropomorphic construction made of various materials intended to mimic the radiological and chemical properties of the human body for the purposes of testing and calibrating radiological devices.)

Estimates of reliability and precision have been limited by concern about the amounts of radiation experienced by persons undergoing repeated neutron bombardment. I have not found a detailed, comprehensive treatment of the radiation hazards associated with in vivo neutron activation analysis. The greater part of the radiation hazard has been attributed to the neutrons rather than the induced radiation. The dose for a single examination for any or all of the elements measured in clinical investigations seems to fall within World Health Organization guidelines for exposures of individual members of the general public [675;676].

Ma and collaborators measured total body calcium, chloride, sodium, phosphorous, nitrogen, and carbon three times in 16 weeks by in vitro neutron activation analysis in 5 weight-stable AIDS patients. Agreements of repeated measurements were gratifying except for total body carbon. The cause for this is unclear but may be a consequence of very small fat deposits in these AIDS patients and a 16 week interval during which the repeated measurements were made [677].

An ability to measure carbon by *in vivo* neutron activation analysis opens some very appealing avenues in the study of human body composition. It offers the possibility of escaping a cruel mathematical necessity in the estimation of fat in the two component models, fat component and fat-free component. To the extent that the fat-free component is over or underestimated, the fat component will be reciprocally under or over estimated. Error in the estimation of the fat-free component is inevitable as a consequence of the assumptions of constancy in it, constant specific density in densitometry, constant concentration of water in the water-based estimate, constant concentration of potassium in the potassium-based estimate. It is *prima facie* unlikely that in all people at all times the specific density, or the concentration of water, or the concentration of potassium in the fat-free component is constant and numerous studies indicate the erroneousness of these assumptions.

Neutron activation analysis depends for quantitation of atoms of body constituents upon measurement of x-rays (γ rays) emitted by excited atoms during decay to a stable state. Atoms are excited by a constant flux of neutrons of known constant intensity.

Presented below is information describing measurement of ^{23}Na as a model of neutron activation analysis of the various substances which can be similarly measured.

The decay scheme for sodium can be understood by conventional notation:

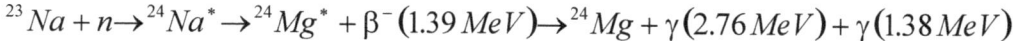

$$^{23}Na + n \rightarrow {}^{24}Na^* \rightarrow {}^{24}Mg^* + \beta^- (1.39\,MeV) \rightarrow {}^{24}Mg + \gamma(2.76\,MeV) + \gamma(1.38\,MeV)$$

in which:

^{23}Na = the predominant naturally occurring isotope of sodium

n = neutron

$^{24}Na^*$ = excited ^{24}Na

$^{24}Mg^*$ = excited ^{24}Mg

β^- *(1.39 MeV)* = negative electron, beta ray, of energy 1.39 *MeV*

^{24}Mg = stable magnesium -24, the predominant naturally occurring isotope

γ *(2.76 MeV)* = gamma ray, X-ray, of energy 2.76 *MeV*

γ *(1.38 MeV)* = gamma ray, X-ray, of energy 1.38 *MeV*

MeV = million electron Volts

Measurement of the quantity of 2.76 *MeV* gamma radiation indexes the amount of ^{24}Na formed which in the presence of a constant neutron flux is a measure of the amount of ^{23}Na present.

The ability to measure carbon, nitrogen, calcium, each independently, offers the possibility of estimating total body fat without resort to the variably invalid assumptions of the two component models. There are other assumptions, which, however, are based on variable amounts of chemical data and have a plausibility lacking in the assumptions of two component models. Those assumptions are:

- •In all persons at all times the carbon content of total body fat is equal to the sum of total body carbon minus the carbon content of total body protein and the carbon content of total body bone,

- •In all persons at all times total body fat has an average carbon content of 77% by weight;

- •In all persons at all times protein contains an average 16% by weight nitrogen;

- •In all persons at all times, protein contains an average 53% by weight carbon,

- •In all persons at all times the weight of carbon in bones is an average 5% of the weight of total body calcium.

Although the above assumptions are plausible, and are supported by some data, close examination reveals that they are only useful approximations. The first assumption, that total body carbon is accounted for as carbon of fat, protein, and bone is known to be incorrect for it does not account for carbon of glycogen and other carbohydrates. Glycogen is found principally in heart, liver, and muscle. It is highly variable but small in quantity and not measurable in vivo by any presently available method. Some authors have included a term for glycogen in their calculations, based on very scant data. Many kinds of substances are known to chemists as "fat", e. g. cholesterol, carbon content 84%. The figure for carbon content of 77% is not applicable to all fats but is a good figure for the fat of adipose tissue and therefore an appropriate value. An assumed value of 16% for the nitrogen content of protein has been used by chemists and physiologists for decades but it is known that different proteins have nitrogen contents ranging from 14% to 17%. Probably a value of 16% is acceptable for the total nitrogen content of the total protein of the human body. Analysis of two cadavers gave values for total nitrogen of total protein of 15.8% and 15.6% [674].

Total body fat can be estimated from measurements by neutron activation analysis of total body carbon, total body nitrogen, and total body calcium, utilizing plausible approximating assumptions. The mathematical expression of these relations follows:

$$TBC = C_f + C_{pr} + C_b$$

in which:

TBC = total body carbon

C_f = carbon of total body fat

C_{pr} = carbon of total body protein

C_b = carbon of total body bone

$C_{pr} = 0.53\ TBP$

in which:

TBP = total body protein

$TBP = TBN\ /\ 0.16 = 6.25\ TBN$

in which:

TBN = total body nitrogen

$C_{pr} = 0.53\ (6.25\ TBN) = 3.31\ TBN$

$C_b = 0.05\ TBCa$

in which:

$TBCa$ = total body calcium

$C_f = TBC - (3.31\ TBN + 0.05\ TBCa)$

$TBF = C_f\,/\,0.77 = 1.3\ C_f$

TBF = total body fat

$TBF = 1.3\ TBC - 4.31\ TBN - 0.06\ TBCa$

Predictive Equations relating densitometrically estimated Fat-free component to arrays of variables including impedance have been developed by many authors employing different arrays. An extensively researched pair of equations, one for men and one for women, has been contributed by Segal and her collaborators [678]:

For men: Fat-free component (Densitometry) = 0.00132 Height^2 - 0.04394 Resistance + 0.030520 Weight - 0.1670 Age + 22.6682

For women: Fat-free component (Densitometry) = 0.00108 Height^2 – 0.02090 Resistance + 0.23199 Weight - 0.06777 Age + 14.594

Correct use of multiple regression equations requires understanding of the assumptions which underlie their construction. Firstly, they describe statistical associations, correlations, between the criterion variable, sometimes called the dependent variable, to the left of the equal sign in the equations above, and the predictor variables, sometimes called the independent variables to the right of the equal sign. The correlated criterion variable and the predictor variables may or may not be causally related in addition to being correlated. Secondly, the form of the equation usually reveals an assumption that each descriptor variable has a straight line, i.e. linear relationship to the criterion variable. Thirdly, the usual tests for statistical significance of the coefficients of the variables assume that the variables have a normal, i.e. Gaussian, distribution. In light of the stringency of these assumptions and the difficulty of validating them, confidence in results will be obtained only when such equations are used in populations very similar to that in which the coefficients were derived.

Skin fold measurement as an avenue to indirect estimation of the percentage of body weight which is fat has stimulated multiple efforts to find mathematics to attain at least an approximation of the size of fat deposits. As in other indirect means of estimating body fat, the efforts are compromised by the fact that there is no rigorous, accepted standard to which to compare them. The most commonly employed criterion method has been densitometry. Many procedures have been described but I will elaborate on only one, that of Durnin and Womersley [67] chosen because it seems to be the method most frequently employed by writers in English. In 481 men and women aged 16 to 72 years Durnin and Womersley measured whole body density as previously described and the thickness of four selected skin folds, two on the arm and two on the trunk (triceps, biceps, subscapular and suprailiac). They found that the relationship of the sum of skin fold thicknesses to density was curvilinear. The relation of the log of the sum of skin fold thicknesses to density appeared to be linear. They computed for each gender and five separate age categories the log-linear regression equation which predicted the mean body density. The whole body density was used to compute percentage body fat by the Siri equation. The regression lines had very similar slopes but their intercepts on the density axis declined with age. This finding is consistent with a shift in the proportion of total body fat which is situated subcutaneously or with an age-related alteration of the density of the fat-free mass. There was also a generally lower intercept for women of all ages. Another problem, recognized by the authors is that the log-linear equation may not be the best fit, especially for the very lean and the very adipose, the latter being rather sparsely represented in their population

Total Body Potassium can be measured and the measurement can be the basis of an estimate of total body fat if it is assumed that potassium is confined to the fat-free component of body composition and the concentration of potassium in that component is known. The size of the fat-free component can be calculated by dividing total potassium by the concentration of potassium. Total body fat is body weight less the fat-free component.

The concentration of potassium in the fat-free component was estimated by a variety of means, e.g. simultaneous measurement of total body potassium and total body water by isotope dilution (see **Isotope Dilution** above). Values reported by different investigators, using different techniques in different populations have varied but virtually all agree that the important differences are the result of age, muscular development, gender, degree of adiposity, medications, and diseases of metabolism, and of heart, lungs, liver, and kidneys. The young and the old have lower values than mature adults [679]. Athletes have higher values than sedentary persons, presumably as a consequence of increased muscular development. Males have higher values than females, presumably a consequence of more muscle. The obese have higher values than thin persons, presumably a consequence of greater muscular development resulting from moving heavy deposits of fat [36;680].

Potassium as it naturally occurs consists of three isotopes, ^{39}K (93.1%), ^{40}K (0.0118%), and ^{41}K (6.88%). (^{42}K was produced by radio nuclide techniques at the Oak Ridge, Tennessee facility of the Atomic Energy Commission and is not found in nature.) ^{40}K is radioactive and can, in principle, be quantitated by measuring its radioactivity. Knowing the amount of ^{40}K present in a body, and knowing the percentage of all potassium which is ^{40}K allows easy calculation of the total potassium in a body. Machines for measuring the radioactivity from ^{40}K in a whole human body, sometimes a very large human body, are large, expensive to acquire, and both expensive and complicated to operate. Significant errors are possible, especially in obese persons in whom significant underestimation may occur as a consequence of self-absorption by tissue of the radiation emitted by the ^{40}K. Estimates of body potassium based on ^{40}K measurements are labeled "total body potassium" to distinguish them from estimates labeled "total exchangeable potassium" made by conventional isotope dilution techniques with injected ^{42}K (see below in **APPENDIX 1**).

The outcome of these efforts is that it may be possible roughly to estimate the fat component in healthy people using total body potassium if age- and gender specific parameters which have been developed in the population of interest are used. It is not an ideal method but one which could occasionally be useful if the necessary machinery is available. Total body potassium is readily calculated from the relation: $^{40}K = 0.00018 \times TBK$

in which
^{40}K = potassium-40
TBK = total body potassium
$TBK = {}^{40}K/0.000118$

Total Exchangeable Potassium measurements attracted interest in the years immediately following the end of World War II when the Atomic Energy Commission made available to biomedical investigators an array of radioactive isotopes, including a radioactive isotope of potassium (^{42}K). Much interest was generated for it was recognized that by application of the principles of isotope dilution as described above , it might be possible to measure total body potassium in a manner analogous to measurement of total body water by isotope dilution. It was speculated that the fat-free component might have a constant concentration of potassium. If that speculation were true, the size of the fat-free component could be estimated by dividing the total body potassium by the concentration of potassium in the fat-free component, analogous to the calculation of fat-free component values from total body water. Values for body potassium estimated in this way were labeled Total Exchangeable Potassium.

Experience with ^{42}K was troubled from the outset. It was contaminated with a radioactive substance or substances which were not potassium. The time for mixing with body potassium was prolonged, and variable, about twenty hours in normal persons, making possible a change in the body content by ingestion or by excretion during the time measurement was occurring. The time period during which one-half of the radioactivity disappeared, the radioactive physical half life, 12.4 hours, was short relative to the time required for mixing with body pools of potassium, making necessary the administration of larger-than-desired doses of radiation in order to have enough activity to measure at the time of equilibration with the crude instruments then available,. An essential assumption of measurement by isotope dilution was found to be invalid in that exchange of the radioactive isotope with native potassium was definitely slower in red blood cells, brain and, especially, bone, than in other organs[681]. A fundamental assumption of isotope dilution measurements is that the isotopically-labeled substance mixes equally well with all pools of the substance being measured. Total exchangeable potassium, utilizing a potassium isotope, ^{42}K, may be calculated by the equation:

$$K_e = \frac{^{42}K_i - \,^{42}K_x}{^{42}K_m \Big/ K_m}$$

In which:

K_e = total exchangeable potassium
$^{42}K_i$ = ^{42}K injected
$^{42}K_x$ = excreted ^{42}K
$^{42}K_m$ = ^{42}K measured in a sample of blood serum or urine
K_m = chemically measured potassium in the above sample of serum or urine

The above measurements are to be made at the time of equilibrium.

Amino acids are small nitrogenous molecules which are assembled into the larger molecules called proteins. Proteins are the structural and catalytic elements of cells. Humans require about 20 amino acids to maintain bodily integrity. Eight of the 20, called essential amino acids, cannot be synthesized in the body and must be obtained from dietary sources. They are isoleucine, leucine, lysine, methionine, phenylalanine,threonine, tryptophan and valine. Recommended dietary protein content is 0.36 g/pound body weight (0.8g/kg) for nonpregnant adults, much less than most Americans eat [682;682].

Cohort Study, sometimes called an observational study or longitudinal study, is one in which a representative group of people is selected, who do not have a risk factor e.g. obesity or an outcome of interest , e.g. arthritis. After an interval, usually of years, both those who have developed the risk factor and those who do not are examined for an outcome, e.g. arthritis. If the risk factor precedes the outcome in time, the study provides evidence that the risk factor predisposes to the outcome.

Comorbidities are morbidities simultaneously present with obesity, considered as a morbidity. They are not necessarily causally related to obesity but often seem to be. Examples of comorbidities frequently occurring and believed to be causally related to obesity are diabetes mellitus (see below), hypertension, and dyslipidemia (see below), Other pathologies less clearly related causally to obesity are various cancers, "wear and tear arthritis" i.e. osteoarthritis, dementia, and obstructive sleep apnea (see below).

Chromosomes are 46 thread-like structures (in humans) contained within the nucleus of each cell. They consist of desoxynucleic acid (DNA), containing the genetically transmissible agents, the genes, assorted regulatory elements, and a variety of proteins.

Diabetes mellitus is classified as Type I and Type II. Both types are characterized by increased concentration of glucose (hyperglycemia) in blood. In the instance of Type I the cause is failure of the pancreas to secrete sufficient insulin. In Type II there is initially resistance to the action of insulin, which is to reduce the concentration of glucose in blood, and later in the disease insufficient secretion of insulin. Both types are associated with severe disease of heart, blood vessels, eyes, kidneys and nervous system.

Dumping Syndrome has as its most frequent cause bariatric surgery. It is frequently incapacitating. The patient experiences abdominal pain, flushing, and faintness soon after eating. One to three hours after eating low blood glucose and symptoms of weakness, confusion, perspiration and hunger may occur. The early symptoms are associated with delivery of large particles of incompletely digested food to the small intestine and the later symptomatic hypoglycemia (low blood glucose) results from rapid delivery of carbohydrates to the small intestine stimulating excessive secretion of insulin [683].

Dyslipidemia is a generic expression indicating abnormal concentrations of fat in blood. Commonly measured fats are cholesterol and triglycerides.

Eating Disorders are most frequent in young females, and have obscure causes. The two most common are anorexia nervosa and bulimia. In anorexia nervosa the patient refuses to eat enough to maintain a healthy body weight and has a self-image of overweight or obesity.. It is sometimes fatal. In bulimia, episodic fasting is followed by binge eating followed by self induced vomiting. Casual observers may be unaware of disordered behavior because the patient is able to live an apparently normal life of work and other activities.

Implanted Defibrillators are battery-powered devices surgically implanted in the chest for the purpose of detecting and correcting a life-threatening type of irregular heart beat. Correction is achieved by delivery of precisely calibrated pulses of electricity to the heart.

Insulin is a proteinaceous hormone secreted by an intra-abdominal organ, the pancreas. It suppresses the release of glucose ("aniimal sugar") by the liver, and enhances the utilization of glucose by other organs, especially muscle. It suppresses release of fatty substances into the blood stream by fat cells.

Isotopes are atoms of the same element which have the same chemical properties and react with other elements in a similar manner but differ either by being heavier or by being radioactive. In a simplified model of an atom the central nucleus of an atom consists of protons and neutrons surrounded by peripheral electrons. Isotopes of the element have the same number of protons but differing numbers of neutrons. For example the most common form of carbon is carbon 12 (^{12}C) which has 6 protons and 6 neutrons. There are 6 rare isotopes all of which have 6 protons but varying numbers of neutrons, 4, 5, 7, 8, 9, and 10.

Meta-analysis combines results of multiple independent studies, usually highly selected, and subjects them to usually rigorous statistical treatment.

Metabolic Syndrome has been defined by an agency of the National Institutes of Health as the presence of three or more of the following: large waist circumference, elevated fasting serum triglycerides, depressed serum HDL cholesterol, hypertension, elevated fasting plasma glucose. In addition to these elements there are other measurements in blood and serum [684] which have attracted attention as possible candidates for inclusion in the syndrome:

-Inflammation-
C-reactive protein
fibrinogen
factor VIIIc
cytokines IL-6, IL-10,TNFα
adhesion molecules ICAM-1, VCAM

-Prothrombotics-
PAI-1
D dimer
fibrinopeptide A

-Oxidant Stress-
oxidized LDL-C
conjugated dienes

Obstructive sleep apnea is a disorder in which breathing repeatedly pauses during sleep as a consequence of anatomic peculiarities of the upper respiratory tract. It is associated with daytime sleepiness, fatigue, irritability and hypertension.

Pulmonary Embolism is a process in which blood clots form in veins, usually of the legs, and travel to the lungs, obstructing blood flow. Risk is enhanced by recent trauma, including surgery, cancer, and venous disease. There is associated significant mortality. A variety of medical interventions are available to reduce risk.

REFERENCE LIST

1. Dellavalle RP, Hester EJ, Hellig LF, Drake AL, Kuntzman JW, Graber M, Schilling LM: Going, Going, Gone: Lost Internet References. Science 2003;302:787-788.

2. Mayer J: Genetic, Traumatic and Environmental Factors in the Etiology of Obesity. Physiological Reviews 1953;33:472-509.

3. Mayer J: Inactivity as a major factor in adolescent obesity. Annals of the New York Academy of Sciences 1965;131:502-506.

4. Kuczmarski RJ, Flegal KM, Campbell SM, Johnson CL: Increasing Prevalence of Overweight Among US Adults. JAMA 1994;272:205-211.

5. Lewis CE, Jacobs DRJr, McCreath H, Kiefe CI, Schreiner PJ, Smith DE, Williams OD: Weight gain continues in the 90s: 10-year trends in weight and overweight from the CARDIA study. Coronary Artery Risk Development in Young Adults. American Journal of Epidemiology 2000;151:1172-1181.

6. Ogden CL, Carroll MD, Curtin LR, McDowell MA, Tabak CJ, Flegal KM: Prevalence of Overweight and Obesity in the United States, 1999-2004. JAMA 2006;295:1549-1555.

7. Prentice AM, Jebb SA: Obesity in Britain: gluttony or sloth? British Medical Journal 1995;311:437-439.

8. Bergman KE, Mensink GB: Anthropometric data and obesity. Gesundheitswesen 1999;61:S115-S120.

9. Flegal KM: The obesity epidemic in children and adults: current evidence and research issues. Medicine and Science in Sports and Exercise 1999;31:S509-S514.

10. WHO Media centre. Obesity and overweight. 2006.

11. Flegal KM, Carroll MD, Ogden CL, Curtin LR: Prevalence and Trends in Obesity Among US Adults, 1999-2008. JAMA 2010;303:235-241.

12. Bessesen DH: Update on Obesity. Journal of Clinical Endocrinology and Metabolism 2008;93:2027-2034.

13. Ford ES, Mokdad AH: Epidemiology of obesity in the Western Hemisphere. Journal of Clinical Endocrinology and Metabolism 2008;93:S1-S8.

14. Wang Y, Monteiro C, Popkin BM: Trends of obesity and underweight in older children and addolescents in the United States, Brazil, China, and Russia. American Journal of Clinical Nutrition 2002;75:971-977.

15. Thorpe KE, Florence CS, Howard DH, Joski P: The Impact of Obesity on Rising Medical Spending. Health Affairs 2004;23:480-486.

16. Food and Agriculture Organization of the United Nations. The State of Food Insecurity in the World 2001. 2001. Ref Type: Electronic Citation

17. Lupien JR: Confusing Food and Obesity. Science 2003;300:1091.

18. Behnke AR, Osserman EF, Welham WC: Lean Body Mass: its Clinical Significance and Estimation from Excess Fat and Total Body Water Determinations. Archives of Internal Medicine 1953;91:585-601.

19. Widdowson EM: Chemical Analysis of the Body; in Brozek J (ed): Human Body Composition. New York 22, N.Y., Pergamon Press Inc., 1965 pp 31-47.

20. Prentice TC, Siri W, Berlin NI, Hyde GM, Parsons RJ, Joiner EE, Lawrence JH: Studies of Total Body Water with Tritium. Journal of Clinical Investigation 1952;31:412-418.

21. Brunton JA, Bayley HS, Atkinson SA: Validation and application of dual-energy x-ray absorptiometry to measure bone mass and body composition in small infants. American Journal of Clinical Nutrition 1993;58:839-845.

22. Kohrt WM: Preliminary evidence that DEXA provides an accurate assessment of body composition. Journal of Applied Physiology 1998;84:372-377.

23. Mitchell AD, Conway JM, Potts WJ: Body composition analysis of pigs by dual-energy X-ray absorptiometry. Journal of Animal Science 1996;74:2663-2671.

24. Mitchell AD, Conway JM, Scholz AM: Incremental Changes in Total and Regional Body Composition of Growing Pigs Measured by Dual-energy X-ray Absorptiometry. Growth,Development & Aging 1996;60:95-105.

25. Mitchell AD, Scholz AM, Conway JM: Body composition analysis of small pigs by dual-energy x-ray absorptiometry. Journal of Animal Science 1998;76:2392-2398.

26. Picaud J-C, Rigo J, Nyamugabo K, Milet J, Senterre J: Evaluation of dual-energy X-ray absorptiometry for body-composition assessments in piglets and term human neonates. American Journal of Clinical Nutrition 1996;63:157-163.

27. Pintauro SJ, Nagy T, Duthie CM, Goran MI: Cross-calibration of fat and lean measurements by dual-energy X-ray absorptiometry to pig carcass analysis in the pediatric body weight range. American Journal of Clinical Nutrition 1996;63:293-298.

28. Roubenoff R, Kehayias J, Dawson-Hughes B, Heymsfield SB: Use of dual-energy x-ray absorptiometry in body composition studies: not yet a "gold standard". American Journal of Clinical Nutrition 1993;58:589-591.

29. Svendsen OL, Haarbo J, Hassager C, Christiansen C: Accuracy of measurements of body composition by dual-energy x-ray absorptiometry in vivo. American Journal of Clinical Nutrition 1993;57:605-608.

30. Baumgartner RN, Heymsfield SB, Lichtman S, Wang J, Pierson JrRN: Body composition in elderly people: effect of criterion estimates on predictive equations. American Journal of Clinical Nutrition 1991;53:1345-1353.

31. Fuller NJ, Jebb SA, Laskey MA, Coward WA, Elia M: Four-component model for the assessment of body composition in humans: comparison with alternative methods, and evaluation of the density and hydration of the fat-free mass. Clinical Science 1992;82:687-693.

32. Heymsfield SB, Lichtman S, Baumgartner RN, Wang J, Kamen Y, Aliprantis A, Pierson JrRN: Body composition of humans:comparison of two improved four-compartment models that differ in expense, technical complexity, and radiation exposure. American Journal of Clinical Nutrition 1990;52:52-58.

33. Fuller NJ, Sawyer MB, Elia M: Comparative Evaluation of Body Composition Methods and Predictions, and Calculation of Density and Hydration of Fat-free Mass, in Obese Women. International Journal of Obesity 1994;18:503-512.

34. Fuller NJ, Elia M: Calculation of body fat in the obese by Siri's formula. European Journal of Clinical Nutrition 1990;44:165-166.

35. Keys A, Brozek J: Body Fat in Adult Man. Physiological Reviews 1953;33:245-325.

36. Hendel HW, Gotfredsen A, Andersen T, Højgaard L, Hilsted J: Body composition during weight loss in obese patients estimated by dual energy X-ray absorptiometry and by total body potassium. International Journal of Obesity 1996;20:1111-1119.

37. Bengtsson B-À, Edèn S, Lönn L, Kvist H, Stokland A, Lindstedt G, Bosaeus I, Tölli J, Sjöström L, Isaksson OG: Treatment of Adults with Growth Hormone (GH) Deficiency with Recombinant Human GH. Journal of Clinical Endocrinology and Metabolism 1993;76:309-317.

38. Hansen TB, Vahl N, Jørgensen JOL, Christiansen JS, Hagen C: Whole body and regional soft tissue changes in growth hormone deficient adults after one year of growth hormone treatment: a double-blind, randomized, placebo-controlled study. Clinical Endocrinology 1995;43:689-686.

39. Jørgensen JOL, Vahl N, Hansen TB, Thuesen L, Hagen C, Christiansen JS: Growth Hormone versus Placebo Treatment for One Year in Growth Hormone Deficient Adults: Increase in Exercise Capacity and Normalization of Body Composition. Clinical Endocrinology 1996;45:681-688.

40. Al-Shoumer KAS, Page B, Thomas E, Murphy M, Beshyah SA, Johnston DG: Effects of Four Years' Treatment with Biosynthetic Human Growth Hormone (GH) on Body Composition in GH-Deficient Hypopituitary Adults. European Journal of Endocrinology 1996;135:559-567.

41. Johannsson G, Mårin P, Ottosson M, Stenlöf K, Björntorp P, Bengtsson B-À: Growth Hormone Treatment of Abdominally Obese Men Reduces Abdominal Fat Mass, Improves Glucose and Lipoprotein Metabolism, and Reduces Diastolic Blood Pressure. Journal of Clinical Endocrinology and Metabolism 1997;82:727-734.

42. Richelsen B, Pedersen SB, Børglum JD, Møller-Pedersen T, Jørgensen J, Jørgensen JO: Growth hormone treatment of obese women for 5 wk: effect on body composition and adipose LPL activity. American Journal of Physiology 1994;266:E211-E216.

43. Svensson J, Jansson J-O, Murphy G, Wyss D, Krupa D, Cerchio K, Polvino W, Gertz B, Bosaeus I, Sjöström L, Bengtsson B-À: Two-Month Treatment of Obese Subjects with the Oral Growth Hormone (GH) Secretagogue MK-677 Increases GH Secretion, Fat-Free Mass, and Energy Expenditure. Journal of Clinical Endocrinology and Metabolism 1998;83:362-369.

44. Thompson JL, Butterfield GE, Gylfadottir UK, Yesavage J, Marcus R, Hintz RL, Pearman A, Hoffman AR: Effects of Human Growth Hormone, Insulin-Like Growth Factor I, and Diet and Exercise on Body Composition of Obese Postmenopausal Women. Journal of Clinical Endocrinology and Metabolism 1998;83:1477-1484.

45. Tomlinson JW, Crabtree N, Clark PMS, Holder G, Toogood AA, Shackleton CHL, Stewart PM: Low-Dose Growth Hormone Inhibits 11β–Hydroxysteroid Dehydrogenase Type 1 but Has No Effect upon Fat Mass in Patientrs withh Simple Obesity. Journal of Clinical Endocrinology and Metabolism 2003;88:2113-2118.

46. Rico H, Revilla M, Villa LF, Ruiz-Contreras D, Hernandez ER, de Buergo MA: The Four-Compartment Models in Body Composition: Data from a Study With Dual-Energy X-Ray Absorptiometry and Near-Infrared Inteeractance on 815 Normal Subjects. Metabolism 1994;43:417-422.

47. Hassager C, Gotfredsen A, Jensen J, Christiansen C: Prediction of Body Composition by Age, Height, Weight, and Skinfold Thickness in Normal Adults. Metabolism 1986;35:1081-1084.

48. Keys A, Fidanza F, Karvonen MJ, Kimura N, Taylor HL: INDICES OF RELATIVE WEIGHT AND OBESITY. Journal of Chronic Disease 1972;25:329-343.

49. Billewicz WZ, Kemsley WFF, Thomson AM: INDICES OF ADIPOSITY. British Journal of preventive and social Medicine 1962;16:183-188.

50. Cali AMG, Caprio S: Obesity in Children and Adolescents. Journal of Clinical Endocrinology and Metabolism 2008;93:531-535.

51. Cole TJ, Bellizi MC, Flegal KM, Dietz WH: Establishing a standard definition for child overweight and obesity worldwide: international survey. BMJ 2000;320:1-6.

52. Allison DB, Paultre F, Poehlman ET, Heymsfield SB: Statistical considerations regarding the use of ratios to adjust data. International Journal of Obesity 1995;19:644-652.

53. Goran MI, Allison DB, Poehlman ET: Issues relating to normalization of body fat content in men and women. International Journal of Obesity 1995;1995:638-643.

54. Bagust A, Walley T: An alternative to body mass index for standardizing body weight for stature. Quarterly Journal of Medicine 2000;93:589-596.

55.Deurenberg P, van der Kooy K, Hulshof T, Evers P: Body mass index as a measure of body fatness in the elderly. European Journal of Clinical Nutrition 1989;43:231-236.

56. Elia M, Parkinson SA, Diaz EO: Evaluation of near infra-red interactance as a method for predicting body composition. European Journal of Clinical Nutrition 1990;44:113-121.

57. Pierson JrRN, Wang J, Heysmfield S, Russell-Aulet M, Mazariegos M, Tierney M, Smith R, Thornton JC, Kehayias J, Weber DA, Dilmanian FA: Measuring Body Fat:Calibrating the Rulers. Intermethod Comparisons in 389 Normal Caucasian Subjects. American Journal of Physiology 1991;261:E103-E108.

58. Pollock ML, Jackson AS: Research progress in validation of clinical methods of assessing body composition. Medicine and Science in Sports and Exercise 1984;16:606-613.

59. Pullicino E, Coward WA, Stubbs RJ, Elia M: Bedside and Field Methods for Assessing Body Composition: Comparison with the Deuterium Dilution Technique. European Journal of Clinical Nutrition 1990;44:753-762.

60. Roche AF, Siervogel RM, Chumlea WC, Webb P: Grading body fatness from limited anthropometric data. American Journal of Clinical Nutrition 1981;34:2831-2838.

61. Ryde SJS, Thomas DW, Birks JL, Ali PA, Saunders NH, Al-Zeibak S, Morgan WD: Assessment of Body Fat: a Comparison of Techniques; in Ellis KJ, Eastman JD (eds): Human Body Composition. New York, Plenum Press, 1993 pp 59-62.

62. Smalley KJ, Knerr AN, Kendrick ZV, Colliver JA, Owen OE: Reassessment of body mass indices. American Journal of Clinical Nutrition 1990;52:405-408.

63. Pietrobelli A, Heymsfield SB: Body mass index as a measure of adiposity among children and adolescents: a validation study. Journal of Pediatrics 1998;132:204-210.

64. Sinning WE: Body composition assessment of college wrestlers. Medicine and Science in Sports 1974;6:139-145.

65. Wang J, Thornton J, Russell M, Burastero S, Heymsfield SB, Pierson JrRN: Asians have lower body mass index (BMI) but higher percent body fat than do whites: comparisons of anthropometric measurements. American Journal of Clinical Nutrition 1994;60:23-28.

66. Kelly, T. L., Wilson, K. E., and Heymsfield, S. B. Dual Energy X-Ray Absorptiometry Body Composition Reference Values from NHANES. 2009.

67. Durnin JVGA, Womersley J: Body fat assessed from total body density and its estimation from skinfold thickness: measurements on 481 men and women aged from 16 to 72 years. British Journal of Nutrition 1974;32:77-97.

68. Strauss MB: Familiar Medical Quotations, ed first. Boston, Little, Brown and Company, 1968.

69. Bruch H: The Importance of Overweight, ed 1. New York, W. W. Norton & Company Inc., 1957.

70. Forbes G: The Great Denial. Nutrition Reviews 1967;25:353-355.

71. Rubin TI: Forever Thin. New York, New York, Gramercy Publishing Company, 1970.

72.Rand C, Stunkard AJ: Obesity and Psychoanalysis. American Journal of Psychiatry 1978;135:547-551.

73. Rand C, Stunkard AJ: Obesity and psychoanalysis: treatment and four-year follow-up. American Journal of Psychiatry 1983;140:1140-1149.

74. Orbach S: Fat is a Feminist Issue. 95 Madison Avenue, New York, New York 10016, Paddington Press Ltd., 1978.

75. Crisp AH, McGuiness B: Jolly fat: relation between obesity and psychoneurosis in general population. British Medical Journal 1976;3:7-9.

76. Hallstrom T, Noppa H: Obesity in women in relation to mental illness, social factors and personality traits. Journal of Psychosomatic Research 1981;25:75-82.

77. Kittell M, Rustin RM, Dramaix M, de Backer G, Kornitzer M: Psycho-biological correlates of moderate overweight in an industrial population. Journal of Psychosomatic Research 1978;22:145.

78. Sallade J: A comparison of the psychological adjustment of obese vs. nonobese children. Journal of Psychosomatic Research 1973;17:89-96.

79. Silverstone JT: Psychosocial aspects of obesity. Proceedings of the Royal Society of Medicine 1968;61:371-375.

80. Stewart AL, Brook AL: Effects of being overweight. American Journal of Public Health 1983;73:171-178.

81. McLaren L, Beck CA, Patten SB, Fick GH, Adair CE: The relationship between body mass index and mental health. A population based study of the effects of definition of mental health. Social Psychiatry and Psychiatric Epidemiology 2008;43:63-71.

82. Petry NM, Barry D, Pietrzak RH, Wagner JA: Overweight and obesity are associated with psychiatric disordes: results from the Naational Epidemiologic Survey on Alcohol and Related Conditions. Psychosomatic Medicine 2008;70:288-297.

83. Simon GE, Von Korff M, Saunders K, Miglioretti DL, Crane PK, van Belle G, Kessler RC: Association between Obesity and Psychiatric Disorders in the US Adult Population. Archives of General Psychiatry 2006;63:824-830.

84. Kivimäki M, Batty GD, Singh-Manoux A, Nabi H, Sabia S, Tabak AG, Akbaraly TN, Vahtera J, Marmot MG, Jokela M: Association between common mental disorder and obesity over the adult life course. British Journal of Psychiatry 2009;195:149-155.

85. Dixon JB, Dixon ME, O'Brien PE: Depression in Association with Severe Obesity. Archives of Internal Medicine 2003;163:2058-2065.

86. Mokhtar N, Elati J, Chabir R, Bour A, Elkari K, Schlossman NP, Caballero B, Aguenaou H: Diet Culture and Obesity in Northern Africa. Journal of Nutrition 2001;131:887S-892S.

87. Fallon AE, Rozin P: Sex Differences in Perceptions of Desirable Body Shapes. Journal of Abnormal Psychology 1985;1985:102-105.

88. Misra A, Khurana L: Obesity and the Metabolic Syndrome in Developing Countries. Journal of Clinical Endocrinology and Metabolism 2008;93:S9-S30.

89. Nielsen SJ, Popkin BM: Patterns and trends in food portion sizes 1977-1998. JAMA 2003;289:450-453.

90. Nestle M: food politics, ed First. Berkeley and Los Angeles, California, University of California Press, 2002.

91. Critser G: FAT LAND, ed First. Boston and New York, Houghton Mifflin Company, 2003.

92. Johnson-Down L, O'Loughlin J, Koski KG, Gray-Donald K: High Prevalence of Obesity in Low Income and Multiethnic Schoolchildren: A Diet and Physical Activity Assessment. Journal of Nutrition 1997;127:2310-2315.

93. Ramsey PW, Glenn LL: Obesity and Health Status in Rural, Urban, and Suburban Southern Women. Southern Medical Journal 2002;95:666-671.

94. Drewnowski A, Specter SE: Poverty and obesity: the role of energy density and energy costs. American Journal of Clinical Nutrition 2004;79:6-16.

95. Pereira MA, Kartashov AI, Ebbeling CB, Van Horn L, Slattery ML, Jacobs DRJr, Ludwig DS: Fast-food habits, weight gain, and insulin resistance (the CARDIA study): 15-year prospective analysis. Lancet 2005;365:36-42.

96. Spence, J. C., Cutumisu, N., Edwards, J., Raine, K. D., and Smoyer-Tomic, K. S. Relation between local food evironments and obesity among adults. BMC Public Health 9. 2009.

97. Drewnowski A: Fat and Sugar: An Economic Analysis. Journal of Nutrition 2003;133:838S-840S.

98. Glanz K, Basil M, Maibach E, Goldberg J, Snyder D: Why Americans eat what they do: taste, nutrition, cost, convenience, and weight control concerns as influences on food consumption. Journal of the American Dietetic Association 1998;11:1118-1126.

99. Christakis NA, Fowler JH: The Spread of Obesity in a Large Social Network over 32 Years. New England Journal of Medicine 2007;357:370-379.

100. Wieben ED: Primer on Medical Genomics. Mayo Clinic Proceedings 2003;78:580-587.

101. Snyder M, Gerstein M: Defining Genes in the Genomics Era. Science 2003;300:258-260.

102. Blakemore AIF, Froguel P: Is Obesity Our Genetic Legacy? Journal of Clinical Endocrinology and Metabolism 2008;93:S51-S56.

103. Bouchard C, Tremblay A, Després J-P, Nadeau A, Lupien PJ, Thériault G, Dussault J, Moorjani S, Pinault S, Fournier G: The resoonse to long-term overfeeding in identical twins. New England Journal of Medicine 1990;322:1477-1482.

104. Stunkard AJ, Harris JR, Pedersen NL, McClearn GE: The body mass index of twins who have been reared apart. New England Journal of Medicine 1990;322:1483-1487.

105. Bouchard, C. Obesity Gene Map. 2001. Internet Communication.

106. Rankinen T, Perusse L, Weisnagel SJ, Snyder EE, Chagnon YC, Bouchard C: The human obesity gene map: the 2001 update. Obesity Research 2002;10:196-243.

107. Glazier AM, Nadeau JH, Aitman TJ: Finding Genes That Underlie Complex Traits. Science 2002;298:2345-2351.

108. Lewis, T. T., Everson-Rose, S. A., Sternfeld, B., Karavolos, K., Wesley, D., and Powell, L. H. Race, Education, and Weight Change in a Biracial Sample of Women at Midlife. Archives of Internal Medicine 165, 545-551. 2005. Ref Type: Generic

109. Anderson SE, Whitaker RC: Prevalence of obesity among US preschool children in different racial and ethnic groups. Archives of Pediatric and Adolescent Medicine 2009;163:344-348.

110. Hirsch J, Han PW: Cellularity of rat adipose tissue: effects of growth, starvation, and obesity. Journal of Lipid Research 1969;10:77-82.

111. Abbott WGH, Foley JE: Comparison of Body Composition, Adipocyte Size, and Glucose and Insulin Concentrations in Pima Indian and Caucasian Children. Metabolism 1987;36:575-579.

112. Danforth E, Jr.: Failure of adipocyte differentiation causes type II diabetes mellitus? Nature Genetics 2000;26:13.

113. Kawada T, Kamei Y, Sugimoto E: The possibility of active form of vitamins A nd D as suppressors on adipocyte development via ligand-dependent transcriptional regulators. International Journal of Obesity 1996;20:S52-S57.

114. Taveras EM, Rifas-Shiman SL, Belfort MB, Kleinman KP, Oken E, Gillman MW: Weight status in the first 6 months of life and obesity at 3 years of age. Pediatrics 2009;123:1177-1183.

115. Levine JA, Jensen MD, Eberhardt NL, O'Brien TO: Adipocyte Macrophage Colony-stimulating Factor is a Mediator of Adipose Tissue Growth. Journal of Clinical Investigation 1998;101:1557-1564.

116. Strawford A, Antelo F, Christiansen M, Hellerstein MK: Adipose tissue glyceride turnover, de novo lipogenesis, and cell proliferation in humans measured with ^2H_2O. American Journal of Physiology Endocrinology and Metabolism 2004;286:E577-E588.

117. Spalding KL, Arner E, Westermark PO, Bernard S, Buchholz BA, Bergmann O, Blomqvist L, Hoffstedt J, Näslund E, Britton T, Concha H, Hassan M, Rydén M, Frisén J, Arner P: Dynamics of fat cell turnover in humans. Nature 2008;453:783-787.

118. Ribon V, Johnson JH, Camp HS, Saltiel AR: Thiazolidinediones and insulin resistance: Peroxisome proliferator-activated receptor γ activation stimulates expression of the CAP gene. Proceedings of the National Academy of Science 1998;95:14751-14756.

119. Tontonoz P, Hu E, Graves RA, Budavari AI, Spiegelman BM: mPPARγ2: tissue-specific regulator of an adipocyte enhancer. Genes & Development 1994;8:1224-1234.

120. Altshuler D, Hirschhorn JN, Lindgren CM, Vohl MC, Nemesh J, Lane CR, Schaffner SF, Bolk S, Brewer C, Tuomi T, Gaudet D, Hudson TJ, Daly M, Groop L, Lander ES: The common PPARgamma Pro12Ala polymorphism is associated with decreased risk of type 2 diabetes. Nature Genetics 2000;26:76-80.

121. Ek J, Urhammer SA, Sorensen TI, Andersen T, Auwerx J, Pedersen O: Homozygosity of the Pr12Ala variant of the peroxisome proliferator-activated receptor-γ2 (PPAR-γ2):divergent modulating effects on body mass index in obese and lean Caucasian men. Diabetologia 1999;42:892-895.

122. Ringel J, Engeli S, Distler A, Sharma AM: Pro12Ala missense mutation of the peroxisome proliferator activated receptor gamma and diabetes mellitus. Biochemical and Biophysical Research Communications 1999;254:450-453.

123. Beamer BA, Yen C-J, Andersen RE, Muller D, Elahi D, Cheskin LJ, Andres R, Roth J, Shuldiner AR: Association of the Pro12Ala Variant in the Peroxisome Proliferator-Activated Receptor-γ2 Gene with Obesity in two Caucasian Populations. Diabetes 1998;47:1806-1808.

124. Valve R, Sivenius K, Miettinen R, Pihlajamäki J, Rissanen A, Deeb SS, Auwerx J, Uusittupa M, Laakso M: Two Polymorphisms in the Peroxisome Proliferator-Activated Receptor-γ Gene Are Associated wwith Severe Overweight among Obese Women. Journal of Clinical Endocrinology and Metabolism 1999;84:3708-3712.

125. Deeb SS, Fajas L, Nemoto M, Pihlajamäki J, Mykkanen L, Kuusisto J, Laakso M, Fujimoto W, Auwerx J: A Pro12Ala substitution in the human peroxisome proliferator activated receptor γ2 associated with decreased receptor activity, lower body mass index and improved insulin sensitivity. Nature Genetics 1998;20:284-287.

126. Oh EY, Min KM, Chung JH, Min Y-K, Lee M-S, Kim K-W, Lee M-K: Significance of Pro[12]Ala Mutation in Peroxisome Proliferator-Activated Receptor-γ[2] in Korean Diabetic and Obese Subjects. Journal of Clinical Endocrinology and Metabolism 2000;85:1801-1804.

127. Memisoglu A, Hu FB, Hankinson SE, Manson JE, De Vivo I, Willett WC, Hunter DJ: Interaction between a peroxisome-activated receptor γ gene in relation to body mass. Human Molecular Genetics 2003;12:2923-2929.

128. Ristow M, Muller-Wieland D, Pfeiffer A, Krone W, Kahn CR: Obesity associated with a mutation in a genetic regulator of adipocyte differentiation. New England Journal of Medicine 1998;339:953-959.

129. Leong NM, Mignone LI, Newcomb PA, Titus-Ernstoff L, Baron JA, Trentham-Dietz A, Stampfer MJ, Willett WC, Egan KM: Early risk factors in cancer: the relation of birth weight to adult obesity. International Journal of Cancer 2003;103:789-791.

130. Martorell R, Stein AD, Schroeder DG: Early Nutrition and Later Adiposity. Journal of Nutrition 2001;131:874S-880S.

131. Parsons TJ, Power C, Manor O: Fetal and early life growth and body mass index from birth to early adulthood in 1958 British cohort: longitudinal study. British Medical Journal 2001;323:1331-1335.

132. Remacle C, Bieswal F, Reusens B: Programming of obesity and cardiovascular disease. International Journal of Obesity and Related Metabolic Disorders 2004;28S:46S-53S.

133. Stocker CJ, Arch JRS, Cawthorne MA: Fetal origins of insulin resistance and obesity. Proceedings of the Royal Society 2005;64:143-151.

134. Gesta S, Blüher M, Yamamoto Y, Norris AW, Berndt J, Kralisch S, Boucher J, Lewis C, Kahn CR: Evidence for a role of developmental genes in the origin of obesity and body fat distribution. Proceedings of the National Academy of Science 2006;103:6676-6681.

135. Wright CM, Parker L, Lamont D, Craft AW: Implications of childhood obesity for adult health: findings from thousand families cohort study. British Medical Journal 2001;323:1280-1284.

136. Guo SS, Roche AF, Chumlea WC, Gardner JD, Siervogel RM: The predictive value of childhood body mass index values for overweight at age 35 y. American Journal of Clinical Nutrition 1994;59:810-819.

137. Guo SS, Wu W, Chumlea WC, Roche AF: Predicting overweight and obesity in adulthood from body mass index values in childhood and adolescence. American Journal of Clinical Nutrition 2002;76:653-658.

138. Reilly JJ, Methven E, McDowell ZC, Hacking B, Alexander D, Stewart L, Kelnar CJH: Health consequences of obesity. Archives of Diseases of Childhood 2003;88:748-752.

139. Serdula MK, Ivery D, Coates RJ, Freedman DS, Williamson DF, Byers T: Do Obese Children Become Obese Adults? A Review of the Literature. Preventive Medicine 1993;22:167-177.

140. Berenson GS, Srinivsan SR, Bao W, Newman III WP, Tracy RE, Wattigney WA: Association between multiple cardiovascular risk factors and atherosclerosis in children and adults. New England Journal of Medicine 1998;338:1650-1656.

141. Woo KS, Yu CW, Sung RY, Quiao M, Leung SS, Lam CW, Metreweii C, Celermajer DS: Overweight in children is associated with arterial endothelial dysfunction and intima-media thickening. International Journal of Obesity and Related Metabolic Disorders 2004;28:852-857.

142. Baker JL, Olsen LW, Sørensen TIA: Childhood Body-Mass Index and the Risk of Coronary Heart Disease in Adulthood. New England Journal of Medicine 2007;357:2329-2337.

143. Hediger ML, Overpeck MD, Kuczmarski RJ, Ruan WJ: Association Between Infant Breastfeeding and Overweight in Young Children. JAMA 2001;285:2453-2460.

144. Gillman MW, Rifas-Shiman SL, Camargo CAJr, Berkey CS, Frazier AL, Rockett HRH, Field AE, Colditz GA: Risk of Overweight Among Adolescents Who Were Breastfed as Infants. JAMA 2001;285:2461-2467.
145. Harder T, Bergmann R, Kallischnigg G, Plagemann J: Duration of Breastfeeding and Risk of Overweight: A Meta-Analysis. American Journal of Epidemiology 2005;162:1-7.

146. Owen CG, Martin RM, Whincup PH, Smith GD, Cook DG: Effect of Infant Feeding on the Risk of Obesity Across the Life Course: A Quantitative Review of Published Evidence. Pediatrics 2005;115:1367-1377.

147. Victora CG, Barros FC, Lima RC, Horta BL, Wells J: Anthropometry and body composition of 18 year old men according to duration of breast feeding: birth cohort study from Brazil. British Medical Journal 2003;327:901-905.

148. Andersen RE, Crespo CJ, Bartlett SJ, Cheskin LJ, Pratt M: Relationship of physical activity and television watdhing with body weight and level of fatness among children : results from the Third National Health and Nutrition Examination Survey. JAMA 1998;25:938-942.

149. Obarzanek E, Schreiber GB, Crawford PB, Goldman SR, Barrier PM, Frederick MM, Lakatos E: Energy intake and physical activity in relation to indexes of body fat: the National Heart, Lung, and Blood Institute Growth and Health Study. American Journal of Clinical Nutrition 1994;60:15-22.

150. Robinson T: Reducing children's television viewing to prevent obesity: a randomized controlled trial. JAMA 1999;282:1561-1567.

151. Hu FB, Li TY, Colditz GA, Willett WC, Manson JE: Television watching and other sedentary behaviors in relation to risk of obesity and type 2 diabetes mellitus in women. JAMA 2003;289:1785-1791.

152. Newburgh LH: Obesity I. energy metabolism. Physiological Reviews 1944;24:18-31

153. Prentice AM, Black AE, Coward WA, Davies HL, Goldberg GR, Murgatroyd PR, Ashford J, Sawyer M, Whitehead RG: High levels of energy expenditure in obese women. British Medical Journal 1986;292:983-987.

154. Seidell JC, Muller DC, Sorkin JD, Andres R: Fasting respiratory exchange ratio and resting metabolic rate as predictors of weight gain: the Baltimore Longitudinal Study on Aging. International Journal of Obesity 1992;16:667-674.

155. Boothby WM, Sandiford I: Summary of the basal metabolism data on 8,614 subjects with especial reference to the normal standards for the estimation of the basal metabolic rate. Journal of Biological Chemistry 1922;54:783-803.

156. Ravussin E, Lillioja S, Knowler WC, Christin L, Freymond D, Abbott WGH, Boyce V, Howard BV, Bogardus C: Reduced rate of energy expenditure as a risk factor for body-weight gain. New England Journal of Medicine 1988;318:467-472.

157. Roberts SB, Savage J, Coward WA, Chew B, Lucas A: Energy expenditure and intake in infants born to lean and overweight mothers. New England Journal of Medicine 1988;318:461-466.

158. Weinsier RL, Nelson KM, Hensrud DD, Darnell BE, Hunter GR, Schutz Y: Metabolic Predictors of Obesity. Journal of Clinical Investigation 1995;95:980-985.

159. Weinsier RL, Nagy T, Hunter GR, Darnell BE, Hensrud DD, Weiss HL: Do adaptive changes in metabolic rate favor weight regain in weight-reduced individuals? An examination of the set-point theory. American Journal of Clinical Nutrition 2000;72:1088-1094.

160. Wong WW, Butte NF, Ellis KJ, Hergenroeder AC, Hill RB, Stuff JE, Smith EO: Pubertal African-American Girls Expend Less Energy at Rest and During Physical Activity than Caucasian Girls. Journal of Clinical Endocrinology and Metabolism 1999;84:906-911.

161. Pittet P, Chappuis P, Acheson KJ, Techterson Fd, Jéquier E: Thermic effect of glucose in obese subjects studied by direct and indirect calorimetry. British Journal of Nutrition 2000;35:281-292.

162. D'Alessio DA, Kavie EC, Mozzoli MA, Smalley KJ, Polansky M, Kendrick ZV, Owen LR, Bushman MC, Boden G, Owen OE: Thermic effect of food in lean and obese men. Journal of Clinical Investigation 1988;81:1781-1789.

163. Tataranni PA, Larson DE, Snitker S, Ravussin E: Thermic effect of food in humans: methods and results from use of a respiratory chamber. American Journal of Clinical Nutrition 1995;61:1013-1019.

164. Levine JA, Eberhardt NL, Jensen MD: Role of Nonexercise Activity Thermogenesis in Resistance to Fat Gain in Humans. Science 1999;283:212-214.

165. Levine JA, Lanningham-Foster LM, McCrady SK, Krizan AC, Olson LR, Kane PH, Jensen MD, Clark MM: Interindividual Variation in Posture Allocation: Possible Role in Human Obesity. Science 2005;307:584-586.

166. Zurlo F, Ferraro RT, Fontvieille AM, Rising R, Bogardus C, Ravussin E: Spontaneous physical activity and obesity: cross-sectional and longitudinal studies in Pima Indians. American Journal of Physiology 1992;263:E296-E300.

167. Cypess AM, Lehman S, Williams G, Tal I, Rodman D, Goldfine AB, Kuo FC, Palmer EL, Tseng Y-H, Doria A, Kolodny GM, Kahn CR: Identification and Importance of Brown Adipose Tissue in Adult Humans`. New England Journal of Medicine 2009;360:1509-1517.

168. Lichtenbelt WDvM, Vanhommerig JW, Smulders NM, Drossaerts JMAFL, Kemerink GJ, Bouvy ND, Schrauwen P, Teule GJJ: Cold-Activated Brown Adipose Tissue in Healthy Men. New England Journal of Medicine 2009;360:1500-1508.

169. Virtanen KA, Lidell ME, Orava J, Heglind M, Westergren R, Niemi T, Taittonen M, Laine J, Savisto N-J, Enerbäck S, Nuutila P: Functional Brown Adipose Tissue in Healthy Adults. New England Journal of Medicine 2009;360:1518-1525.

170. Cannon B, Nedergaard J: Brown Adipose Tissue: Function and Physiological Significance. Physiological Reviews 2004;84:277-359.

171. Leibel R, Rosenbaum M, Hirsch J: Changes in energy expenditure resulting from altered body weight. New England Journal of Medicine 1995;332:621-628.

172. Bachman ES, Dhillon H, Zhang C-Y, Cinti S, Bianco AC, Kobilka BK, Lowell BB: βAR Signaling Required for Diet-induced Thermogenesis and Obesity Resistance. Science 2002;297:843-845.

173. Tataranni PA, Young JB, Bogardus C, Ravussin E: A low sympathoadrenal activity is associated with body weight gain and development of central adiposity in Pima Indian men. Obesity Research 1997;5:341-347.

174. Weinsier RL, Hunter GR, Heini AF, Goran MI, Sell SM: The Etiology of Obesity: Relative Contribution of Metabolic Factors, Diet, and Physical Activity. American Journal of Medicine 1998;105:145-150.

175. Arnett DK, Xiong B, McGovern PG, Blackburn H, Luepker RV: Secular Trends in Dietary Macronutrient Intake in Minneapolis-St.Paul, Minnesota,1980-1992. American Journal of Epidemiology 2000;152:868-873.

176. Ley RE, Turnbaugh PJ, Klein S, Gordon JL: Microbial ecology: human gut microbes associated with obesity. Nature 2006;444:1022-1023.

177. Bäckhed F, Ding H, Wang T, Hooper LV, Koh GY, Nagy A, Semenkovich CF, Gordon JL: The gut microbiota as an environmental factor that regulates fat storage. Proceedings of the National Academy of Science 2004;101:15718-15723.

178. Kalliomäki M, Collado MC, Salminen S, Isolauri I: Early differences in fecal microbiota composition in children may predict overweight. American Journal of Clinical Nutrition 2008;87:534-538.

179. Stewart JA, Chadwick VS, Murray A: Investigations into the influence of host genetics on the predo inant eubacteria in faecal microflora of children. Journal of Medical Microbiology 2005;54:1239-1242.

180. Turnbaugh PJ, Hamady M, Yatsunenko T, Cantarel BL, Duncan A, Ley RE, Sogin SL, Jones WJ, Roe BA, Affourtit JP, Egholm M, Henrissat B, Heath AC, Knight R, Gordon JI: A core gut microbiome in obese and lean twins. Nature 2009;457:480-484.

181. DiBaise JK, Zhang H, Crowell MD, Krajmalnik-Brown R, Decker GA, Rittman BE: Gut Microbiota and Its Poss blle Relationship With Obesity. Mayo Clinic Proceedings 2008;83:460-469.

182. Kottke TE, Clark MM, Aase LA, Brandel CL, Brekke MJ, Brekke LN, DeBoer SW, Hayes SN, Hoffman RS, Menzel PA, Thomas RJ: Self-reported Weight, Weight Goals, and Weight Control Strategies of a Midwestern Population. Mayo Clinic Proceedings 2002;77:114-121.

183. Zurlo F, Lillioja S, Esposito-del Puente A, Nyomba BL, Raz I, Saad MF, Swinburn BA, Knowler WC, Bogardus C, Ravussin E: Low ratio of fat to carbohydrate oxidation as predictor of weight gain: study of 24-h RQ. American Journal of Physiology 1990;259:E650-E657.

184. Hellerstein MK, Christiansen M, Kaempfer S, Wu K, Reid JS, Mulligan K, Hellerstein NS, Shackleton CHL: Measurement of De Novo Hepatic Lipogenesis in Humans Using Stable Isotopes. Journal of Clinical Investigation 1991;87:1841-1852.

185. Schwarz J-M, Neese RA, Turner S, Dare D, Hellerstein MK: Short-Term Alterations in Carbohydrate Energy Intake in Humans. J Clin Invest 1995;96:2735-2743.

186. McDevitt RM, Bott SJ, Harding M, Coward WA, Bluck LJ, Prentice AM: De novo lipogenesis during controlled overfeeding with sucrose or glucose in lean and obese women. American Journal of Clinical Nutrition 2001;74:737-746.

187. Colberg SR, Simoneau JA, Thaete FL, Kelley DE: Skeletal muscle utilization of free fatty acids in women with visceral obesity. Journal of Clinical Investigation 1995;95:1846-1853.

188. Kim J-K, Hickner RC, Cortwright RL, Dohm GL, Houmard JA: Lipid oxidation is reduced in obese human skeletal muscle. American Journal of Physiology 2000;279:E1039-E1044.

189. Simoneau J-A, Veerkamp JH, Turcotte LP, Kelley DE: Markers of capacity to utilize fatty acids in human skeletal muscle: relation to insulin resistance and obesity and effects of weight loss. FASEB Journal 1999;13:2051-2060.

190. Kelley DE, Goodpaster B, Wing RR, Simoneau J-A: Skeletal muscle fatty acid metabolism in association with insulin resistance, obesity, and weight loss. American Journal of Physiology 1999;277:E1130-E1141.

191. Ruderman NB, Saha AK, Vavvas D, Witters LA: Malonyl-CoA, fuel sensing, and insulin resistance. American Journal of Physiology 1999;276:E1-E18.

192. Longo N, di San Filippo CA, Pasquali M: Disorders of carnitine transport and the carnitine cycle. American Journal of Medical Genetics 2006;142C:77-85.

193. Brown NF, Mullur RS, Subramanian I, Esser V, Bennett MJ, Saudubray JM, Feigenbaum AS, Kobari JA, Macleod PM, McGarry JD, Cohen JC: Molecular characterization of L-CPT I deficiency in six patientxs: insights into the function of the native enzyme. Journal of Lipid Research 2001;42:1134-1142.

194. Prasad C, Johnson JP, Bonnefont JP, Dilling LA, Innes AM, Haworth JC, Beischel L, Thuilier L, Prip-Buus C, Singal R, Thompson JR, Prasad AN, Buist N, Greenberg CR: Hepatic carnitine palmitoyl transferase 1 (CPT1 A) deficiency in North American Hutterites (Canadian and American): evidence for a founder effect and results of a pilot study on a DNA-based newborn screening program. Molecular Genetics and Metabolism 2001;73:55-63.

195. Schutz Y, Tremblay A, Weinsier RL, Nelson KM: Role of fat oxidation in the long-term stabilization of body weight in obese women. American Journal of Clinical Nutrition 1992;55:670-674.

196. Maffeis C, Armellini F, Tato L, Schutz Y: Fat Oxidation and Adiposity in Prepubertal Children: Exogenous versus Endogenous Fat Utilization. Journal of Clinical Endocrinology and Metabolism 1999;84:654-658.

197. Ingalls AM, Dickie MM, Snell GD: OBESE, A new mutation in the house mouse. Journal of Heredity 1950;41:317-318.

198. Coleman DL: Obese and Diabetes: two Mutant Genes Causing Diabetes-Obesity Syndromes in Mice. Diabetologia 1978;14:141-148.

199. Zhang Y, Proenca R, Maffei M, Barone M, Leopold L, Friedman JM: Positional cloning of the mouse obese gene and its human homologue. Nature 1994;372:425-432.

200. Moon BC, Friedman JM: The molecular basis of the obese mutation in ob2J mice. Genomics 1997;42:152-156.

201. Halaas JL, Maffei M, Cohen SL, Chait BT, Rabinowitz D, Lallone RL, Burley SK, Friedman JM: Weight-Reducing Effects of the Plasma Protein Encoded by the obese Gene. Science 1995;269:543-546.

202. Montague CT, Farooql IS, Whitehead JP, Soos MA, Rau H, Wareham NJ, Sewter CP, Digby JE, Mohammed SN, Hurst JA, Cheetham CH, Earley AR, Barnett AH, Prins JB, O'Rahilly S: Congenital leptin deficiency is associated with severe early-onset obesity in humans. Nature 1997;387:903-908.

203. Farooql IS, Jebb SA, Langmack G, Lawrence E, Cheetham CH, Prentice AM, Hughes IA, McCamish MA, O'Rahilly S: Effects of Recombinant Leptin Therapy in a Child with Congenital Leptin Deficiency. New England Journal of Medicine 1999;341:879-884.

204. Farooql IS, Matarese G, Lord GM, Keogh JM, Lawrence E, Agwu C, Sanna V, Jebb SA, Perna F, Fontana S, Lechler RI, DePaoli AM, O'Rahilly S: Beneficial effects of leptin on obesity, T cell hyporesponsiveness, and neuroendocrine/metabolic dysfunction of human congenital leptin deficiency. Journal of Clinical Investigation 2002;110:1093-1103.

205. Williams LB, Fawcett RL, Waechter AS, Zhang P, Kogon BE, Jones R, Inman M, Huse J, Considine RV: Leptin Production in Adipocytes from Morbidly Obese Subjects: Stimulation by Dexamethasone, Inhibition with Troglitazone, and Influence of Gender. Journal of Clinical Endocrinology and Metabolism 2000;85:2678-2684.

206. Clement K, Vaisse C, Lahlou N, Cabrol S, Pelloux V, Cassuto D, Gourmelen M, Dina C, Chambaz J, Lacorte J-M, Basdevant A, Bougnères P, Lebouc Y, Froguel P, Guy-Grand B: A mutation in the human leptin receptor gene causes obesity and pituitary dysfunction. Nature 1998;392:398-401.

207. Minokoshi Y, Kim YB, Peroni OD, Fryer LG, Muller C, Carting D, Kahn BB: Leptin stimulates fatty-acid oxidation by activating AMP-activated protein kinase. Nature 2002;17:339-343.

208. Wong, M-L., Licinio, J., Yildiz, B. O., Mantzoros, C. S., Prolo, P., Kling, M., and Gold, P. W. Simultaneous and Continuous 24-Hour Plasma and Cerebrospinal Fluid Leptin Measurements: Dissociation of Concentrations in Central; and Peripheral Compartments. Journal of Clinical Endocrinology and Metabolism 89, 258-265. 2004.

209. Heymsfield SB, Greenberg AS, Fujioka K, Dixon RM, Kushner R, Hunt T, Lubina JA, Patane J, Self B, Hunt P, McCamish M: Recombinant Leptin for Weight Loss in Obese and Lean Adults. JAMA 1999;282:1568-1576.

210. Farooql IS, Keogh JM, Kamath S, Jones S, Trussell R, Jebb SA, Lip GYH, O'Rahilly S: Partial leptin deficiency and human adiposity. Nature 2001;414:34-35.

211. Löfgren P, Andersson I, Adolfsson B, Leijonhufvud B-M, Hertel K, Hoffstedt J, Arner P: Long-Term Prospective and Controlled Studies Demonstrate Adipose Tissue Hypercellularity and Relative Leptin Deficiency in the Postobese State. Journal of Clinical Endocrinology and Metabolism 2005;90:6207-6213.

212. Hukshorn CJ, Saris WHM, Westerterp-Plantenga MS, Farid AR, Smith FJ, Campfield LA: Weekly Subcutaneous Pegylated Recombinant Native Human Leptin (PEG-OB) Administration in Obese Men. Journal of Clinical Endocrinology and Metabolism 2000;85:4003-4009.

213. Taylor AE, Hubbard J, Anderson EJ: Impact of Binge Eating on Metabolic and Leptin Dynamics in Normal Young Women. Journal of Clinical Endocrinology and Metabolism 1999;84:428-434.

214. Kolaczynski JW, Considine RV, Ohannesian J, Marco C, Opentanova I, Nyce MR, Myint M, Caro JF: Responses of Leptin to Short-Term Fasting and Refeeding in Humans. A Link with Ketogenesis but Not Ketones Themselves. Diabetes 1996;45:1511-1515.

215. Rosenbaum M, Nicolson M, Hirsch J, Murphy E, Chu F, Leibel RE: Effect on Weight Changes on Plasma Leptin Concentrations and Energy Expenditure. Journal of Clinical Endocrinology and Metabolism 1997;82:3647-3654.

216. Chin-Chance C, Polonsky KS, Schoeller DA: Twenty-Four-Hour Leptin Levels Respond to Cumulative Short-Term Energy Imbalance and Predict Subsequent Intake. Journal of Clinical Endocrinology and Metabolism 2000;85:2685-2691.

217. Gibbons A: Oldest Members of Homo sapiens Discovered in Africa. Science 2003;300:1641.

218. Lev-Ran A: Human obesity: an evolutionary approach to understanding our bulging waistline. Diabetes/ Metabolism Research and Reviews 2005;17:347-362.

219. Peppard PE, Young T, Palta M, Dempsey J: Longitudinal Study of Moderate Weight Change and Sleep-Disordered Breathing. JAMA 2000;284:3015-3021.

220. Gotoda T, Scott J, Altman TJ: Molecular screening of the human melanocortin-4 receptor gene: identification of a missense variant showing no association with obesity, plasma glucose, or insulin. Diabetologia 1997;40:976-979.

221. Hainerová I, Larsen LH, Holst B, Finková M, Vojtêch H, Lebl J, Hansen T, Pedersen O: Melanocortin 4 Receptor Mutations in Obese Czech Children: Studies of Prevalence, Phenotype Development, Weight Reduction Response, and Functional Analysis. Journal of Clinical Endocrinology and Metabolism 2007;92:3689-3696.

222. Hinney A, Bettecken T, Tarnow P, Brumm H, Reichwald K, Lichtner P, Scherag A, Nguyen TT, Schlumberger P, Rief W, Vollmert C, Illig T, Wichmann H-E, Schäfer H, Platzer M, Biebermann H, Meitinger T, Hebebrand J: Prevalence, Spectrum, and Functional Characterization of Melanocortin-4 Receptor Gene Mutations in a Representative Population-Based Sample and Obese Adults from Germany. Journal of Clinical Endocrinology and Metabolism 2006;91:1761-1769.

223. Jacobson P, Ukkola O, Rankinen T, Snyder EE, Leon AS, Rao DC, Skinner JS, Wilmore JH, Lönn L, Cowan GS, Jr., Sjöström L, Bouchard C: Melanocortin 4 Receptor Seque4nce Variations are Seldom a Cause of Human Obesity: The Swedish Obese Subjects, the HERITAGE Family Study, and a Memphis Cohort. Journal of Clinical Endocrinology and Metabolism 2002;87:4442-4446.

224. Lubrano-Berthelier C, Dubern B, Lacorte J-M, Picard F, Shapiro A, Zhang S, Bertrais S, Hercberg S, Basdevant A, Clement K, Vaisse C: Melanocortin 4 Receptor Mutations in a Large Cohort of Severely Obese

Adults: Prevalence, Functional Classification, and Lack of Association with Binge Eating. Journal of Clinical Endocrinology and Metabolism 2006;91:1811-1818.

225. Miraglia DGE, Cirillo G, Nigro V, Santoro N, D'Urso L, Raimondo P, Cozzolino D, Scafato D, Perrone L: Low frequency of melanocortin-4 receptor (MC4R) mutations in a Mediterranean population with early-onset obesity. International Journal of Obesity and Related Metabolic Disorders 2002;26:647-651.

226. O'Rahilly S, Farooqi IS, Yeo GSH, Challis BG: Minireview: Human Obesity - Lessons from Monogenic Disorders. Journal of Clinical Endocrinology and Metabolism 2003;144:3757-3764.

227. Cone RD: Haploinsufficiency of the melanocortin-4 receptors: part of a thrifty genotype? Journal of Clinical Investigation 2000;106:185-187.

228. Tao Y-X, Segaloff DL: Functional Analyses of Melanocortin-4 Receptor Mutations Identified from Patients with Binge Eating Disorder and Nonobese or Obese Subjects. Journal of Clinical Endocrinology and Metabolism 2005;90:5632-5638.

229. Jackson RS, Creemers JWM, Ohagi S, Raffin-Sanson M-L, Sanders L, Montague CT, Hutton JC, O'Rahilly S: Obesity and impaired prohormone processing associated with mutations in the human prohormone convertase 1 gene. Nature Genetics 1997;16:303-306.

230. Krude H, Biebermann H, Luck W, Horn R, Brabant G, Gruters A: Severe early-onset obesity, adrenal insufficiency and red hair pigmentation caused by POMC mutations in humans. Nature Genetics 1998;19:155-157.

231. Lee YS, Challis BG, Thompson DA, Yeo GS, Keogh JM, Madonna ME, Wraight V, Sims M, Vatin V, Meyre D, Shield J, Burren C, Ibrahim Z, Swift P, Blackwood A, Hung CC, Wareham NJ, Froquel P, Millhauser GL, O'Rahilly S, Farooqi IS: A POMC variant implicates beta-melanocyte-stimulating hormone in the control of human energy balance. Cell Metabolism 2006;3:135-140.

232. Rankinen T, Zuberi A, Chagnon YC, Weisnagel SJ, Argyropoulos G, Walts B, Pérusse L, Bouchard C: Human Obesity Gene Map. The 2005 Update. Obesity 2006;14:529-644.

233. Willer CJ, Speliotes EK, Loos RJF, Shengxu L, Lindgren CM, Heid IM, Berndt SI, Elliot AL, Jackson AU, Lamina C, Lettre G, Lim N, Lyon HN, McCarroll SA, Papadakis K, Qi L, Randall JC, Roccasecca RM, Sana S, Scheet P, Weedon MN, Wheeler E, Zhao JH, Jacobs LC, Prokopenko I, Soranzo N, Tanaka T, Timpson NJ, Almgren P, Bennett A, Bergman RN, Bingham SA, Bonnycastle LL, Brown M, Burtt NP, Chines P, Coin L, Collins FS, Connell JM, Cooper C, Smith GD, Dennison EM, Deodhar P, Elliot P, Erdos MR, Estrada K, Evans DM, Gianniny L, Gieger C, Gillson CJ, Guiducci C, Hackett R, Hadley D, Hall AS, Havulinna AS, Hebebrand J, Hofman A, Isomaa B, Jacobs KB, Johnson T, Jousilahti P, Jovanovic Z, Khaw K-T, Kraft P, Kuokkanen M, Kuusisto J, Laitinen J, Lakatta EG, Luan J, Luben RN, Mangino M, McArdle WL, Meitinger T, Mulas A, Munroe PB, Narisu N, Ness AR, Northstone K, O'Rahilly S, Purmann C, Rees MG, Ridderstråle M, Ring SM, Rivadeneira F, Ruokonen A, Sandhu MS, Saramies J, Scott LJ, Scuteri A, Silander K, Sims MA, Song J, Stephens J, Stevens S, Stringham HM, Tung YCL, Valle TT, Van Duijn CM, Vimaleswaran KS, Vollenweider P, Waeber G, Wallace C, Watanabe RN, Waterworth DM, Watkins N, Wellcome Trust Case Control Consortium, Witteman JCM, Zeggini E, Zhai G, Zillikens MC, Altshuler D, Caulfield MJ, Chanock SJ, Farooqi IS, Ferrucci L, Guralnik JM, Hattersley AT, Hu FB, Jarvelin M-R, Laakso M, Mooser V, Ong KK, Ouwehand WH, Salomaa V, Samani NJ, Spector TD, Tuomi T, Tuomilehto J, Uda M, Uitterlinden AG, Wareham NJ, Deloukas P, Frayling TM, Groop LC, Hayes RB, Strachan DP, Wichmann H-E, McCarthy MI, Boehnke D, Barroso I, Abecasis GR, Hirschhorn JN: Six new loci associated with body mass index highlight a neuronal influence on body weight regulation. Nature Genetics 2009;41:25-34.

234. Kojima M, Hosoda H, Date Y, Nakazato M, Matsuoka H, Kangawa K: Ghrelin is a growth-hormone-releasing acylated peptide from stomach. Nature 1999;402:656-660.

235. Wren AM, Seal LJ, Cohen MA, Brynes AE, Frost GS, Murphy KG, Dhillo WS, Ghatei MA, Bloom SR: Ghrelin Enhances Appetite and Increases Food Intake in Humans. Journal of Clinical Endocrinology and Metabolism 2001;86:5992-5995.

236. Monteleone, P., Bencivenga, R., Longobardi, N., Serritella, C., and Maj, M. Differential Responses of Circulating Ghrelin to High-Fat or High-CarbohydrateMeal in Healthy Women. Journal of Clinical Endocrinology and Metabolism 88, 5510-5514. 2003.

237. Leidy HJ, Gardner JK, Frye BR, Schuchert MK, Richard EL, Williams NI: Circulating Ghrelin Is Sensitive to Changes in Body Weight during a Diet and Exercise Program in Normal-Weight Young Women. Journal of Clinical Endocrinology and Metabolism 2004;89:2659-2664.

238. Tschöp M, Weyer C, Tataranni PA, Devanarayan V, Ravussin E, Heiman M: Circulating Ghrelin Levels Are Decreased in Human Obesity. Diabetes 2001;50:707-709.

239. Adrian TE, Ferri GL, Bacarese-Hamilton AJ, Fuessl HS, Polak JM, Bloom SR: Human distribution and release of a putative new gut hormone, peptide YY. Gastroenterology 1985;89:1070-1077.

240. Adrian TE, Bloom SR, Bryant MG, Polak JM, Heitz PH, Barnes AJ: Distribution and release of human pancreatic polypeptide. Gut 1976;17:940-944.

241. Batterham RL, Cohen MA, Ellis SM, Le Roux CW, Withers DJ, Frost GS, Ghatei MA, Bloom SR: Inhibition of food intake in obese subjects by peptide YY3-36. New England Journal of Medicine 2003;349:926-928.

242. Batterham RL, Cowley MA, Small CJ, Herzog H, Cohen MA, Dakin CL, Wren AM, Brynes AE, Low MJ, Ghatei MA, Cone RD, Bloom SR: Gut hormone PYY(3-36) physiologically inhibits food intake. Nature 2002;418:595-597.

243. Batterham RL, Le Roux CW, Cohen MA, Park AJ, Ellis SM, Patterson M, Frost GS, Ghatei MA, Bloom SR: Pancreatic polypeptide reduces appetite and food intake in humans. Journal of Clinical Endocrinology and Metabolism 2003;88:3989-3992.

244. Glaser B, Zoghlin G, Pienta K, Vinik A: Pancreatic polypeptide response to secretin in obesity: effects of glucose intolerance. Hormone and Metabolic Research 1988;20:288-292.

245. Le Quellec A, Kervran A, Blache P, Clurans AJ, Bataille D: Oxyntomodulin-like immunoreactivity: diurnal profile of a new potential enterogastrone. Journal of Clinical Endocrinology and Metabolism 1992;74:1405-1409.

246. Cohen MA, Ellis SM, Le Roux CW, Batterham RL, Park A, Patterson M, Frost GS, Ghatei MA, Bloom SR: Oxyntomodulin Suppresses Appetite and Reduces Food Intake in Humans. Journal of Clinical Endocrinology and Metabolism 2003;88:4696-4701.

247. Verdich C, Toubro S, Buemann B, Madsen JL, Holst JJ, Astrup A: the role pf postprandial releases of insulin and incretin hormones in meal-induced satiet-effect of obesity and weight reduction. International Journal of Obesity 2001;25:1206-1214.

248. Gutzmiller J-P, Göke B, Drewe J, Hilldebrand P, Ketterer S, Handschin D, Winterhalder R, Conen D, Beglinder C: Glucagon-like peptide-1 : apotent regulator of food intake in humans. Gut 1999;44:81-86.

249. Naslund E, Barkeling B, King N, Gutniak M, Blundell JE, Holst JJ, Rossner S, Hellstrom PM: Energy intake and appetite are suppressed by glucagon-like peptide-1 (GLP-1) in obese men. International Journal of Obesity and Related Metabolic Disorders 1999;23:304-311.

250. Lieverse RJ, Jansen JB, Masclee AA, Rovati LC, Lamers CB: Effect of a low dose of intraduodenal fat on satiety in humans: studies using the type A cholecystokinin receptor antagonist loxiglumide. Gut 1994;35:501-505.

251. Lieverse RJ, Jansen JB, Masclee AA, Lamers CB: Satiety effects of a physiological dose of cholecystokinin in humans. Gut 1995;36:176-179.
252. Muurahainen N, Kissileff HR, Derogatis AJ, Pi-Sunyer FX: Effects of cholecystokinin-octapeptide (CCK-8) on food intake and gastric emptying in man. Physiology & Behavior 1988;44:645-649.

253. Moran TH, Schwartz GJ: Neurobiology of cholecystokinin. Critical Reviews in Neurobiology 1994;9:1-28.

254. Schwartz MW: Staying Slim with Insulin in Mind. Science 2000;289:2066-2067.

255. Brüning JC, Gautam D, Burks DJ, Gillette J, Schubert M, Orban PC, Klein R, Krone W, Müller-Wieland D, Kahn CR: Role of Brain Insulin Receptor in Control of Body Weight and Reproduction. Science 2000;289:2122-2125.

256. Obici S, Feng Z, Karkanias G, Baskin DG, Rossetti L: Decreasing hypothalamic insulin receptors causes hyperphagia and insulin resistance in rats. Nature Neuroscience 2002;5:566-572.

257. Air EL, Strowski MZ, Benoit SC, Conarello S, Salituro GM, Guan XM, Liu K, Woods SC, Zhang BB: Small molecule insulinmimetics reduce food intake and body weight and prevent development of obesity. Nature Medicine 2002;8:179-183.

258. Schwartz GJ: The role of gastrointestinal vagal afferents in the control of food intake: current prospects. Nutrition 2000;16:866-873.

259. Foster-Schubert KE, Overduin O, Prudom CE, Liu J, Callahan HS, Gaylinn BD, Thorner MO, Cummings DE: Acyl and Total Ghrelin are Suppressed Strongly by Ingested Proteins, Weakly by Lipids, and Biphasically by Carbohydrates. Journal of Clinical Endocrinology and Metabolism 2008;93:1971-1979.

260. Schwartz MW, Baskin DG, Kalyalla KJ, Woods SC: Model for the regulation of energy balance and adiposity by the central nervous system. American Journal of Clinical Nutrition 1999;69:584-596.

261. Goldstone AP, Brynes AE, Thomas EL, Bell JD, Frost G, Holland A, Ghatei MA, Bloom SR: Resting metabolic rate, plasma leptin concentrations, leptin receptor expression, and adipose tissue measured by whole-body magnetic resonance imaging in women with Prader-Willi syndrome. American Journal of Clinical Nutrition 2002;75:468-475.

262. Haqq AM, Farooqi IS, O'Rahilly S, Stadler DD, Rosenfeld RG, Pratt KL, LaFranchi SH, Purnell JQ: Serum Ghrellin Levels Are Inversely Correlated with Body Mass Index, Age, and Insulin Concentrations in Normal Children and Are Markedly Increased in Prader-Willi Syndrome. Journal of Clinical Endocrinology and Metabolism 2003;88:174-178.

263. Zipf WB, O'Dorisio TM, Cataland S, Sotos J: Blunted pancreatic polypeptide responses in children with obesity of Prader-Willi syndrome. Journal of Clinical Endocrinology and Metabolism 1981;52:1264-1266.

264. Berntson GG, Zipf WB, O'Dorisio TM, Hoffman JA, Chance RE: Pancreatic Polypeptide Infusions Reduce Food Intake in Prader-Willi Syndrome. Peptides 1993;14:497-503.

265. Greenswag LR: Adults with Prader-Willi syndrome: a survey of 232 cases. Developmental Medicine and Child Neurology 1987;29:145-152.

266. Vogels A, Fryns JP: The Prader-Willi syndrome and the Angelman syndrome. Genetic Counseling 2002;13:385-396.

267. Woods MO, Young TL, Parfrey PS, Hefferton D, Green JS, Davidson WS: Genetic heterogeneity of Bardet-Biedl syndrome in a distinct Canadian population: evidence for a fifth locus. Genomics 1999;55:2-9.

268. Katsanis N, Ansley SJ, Badano JL, Eichers ER, Lewis RA, Hoskins BE, Scrambler PJ, Davidson WS, Beales PL, Lupski JR: Triallelic Inheritance in Bardet-Biedl Syndome, a Mendelian Recessive Disorder. Science 2001;293:2256-2259.

269. Fan Y, Esmail MA, Ansley SJ, Blacque OE, Boroevich K, Ross AJ, Moore SJ, Badano JL, May-Simera H, Compton DS, Green JS, Lewis RA, van Haeist MM, Parfrey PS, Baillie DL, Beales PL, Katsanis N, Davidson WS, Leroux MR: Mutations in a member of the RAS superfamily of small GTP-binding proteins causes Bardet-Biedl syndrome. Nature Genetics 2004;36:989-993.

270. Kok SW, Meinders S, Overeem S, Lammers GJ, Roelfsema F, Frölich M: Reduction of Plasma Leptin Levels and Loss of Its Circadian Rhymicity in Hypocretin (Orexin)-Deficient Narcoleptic Humans. Journal of Clinical Endocrinology and Metabolism 2002;87:805-809.

271. Lubkin M, Stricker-Krongrad A: Independent feeding and metabolic actions of orexins in mice. Biochemical and Biophysical Research Communications 1998;253:241-245.

272. Vague J: La differénciation sexuelle, facteur determinant des formes de l'obésité. La Presse Médicale 1947;55:339-340.

273. Vague J: The degree of masculine differentiation of the obesities, a factor determining predisposition to diabetes, atherosclerosis, gout, and uric calculous disease. American Journal of Clinical Nutrition 1956;4:20-34.

274. Bujalska IJ, Kumar S, Stewart PM: Does central obesity reflect "Cushing's disease of the omentum"? Lancet 1997;349:1210-1213.

275. Hauner H, Entenmann G, Wabitsch M, Gaillard D, Ailhaud G, Negrel R, Pfeiffer EF: Promoting effect of glucocorticoids on the differentiation of human adipocyte precursor cells cultured in a chemically defined medium. Journal of Clinical Investigation 1989;84:1663-1670.

276. Masuzaki H, Paterson J, Shinyama H, Morton NM, Mullins JJ, Seckl JR, Flier JS: A Transgenic Model of Visceral Obesity and the Metabolic Syndrome. Science 2001;294:2166-2170.

277. Montague CT, O'Rahilly S: The Perils of Portliness. Diabetes 2000;49:883-888.

278. Kvist H, Chowdhury B, Grangård U, Tylén U, Sjöström L: Total and visceral adipose-tissue volumes derived from measurements with computed tomography in adult men and women: predictive equations. American Journal of Clinical Nutrition 1988;48:1351-1361.

279. Mårin P, Holmäng S, Jönsson L, Sjöström L, Kvist H, Holm G, Lindstedt G, Björntorp P: The effects of testosterone treatment on body composition and metabolism in middle-aged obese men. International Journal of Obesity 1992;16:991-997.

280. Seidell JC, Björntorp P, Sjöström L, Kvist H, Sannerstedt R: Visceral fat accumulation in men is positively associcted with insulin, glucose, and C-peptide levels, but negatively with testosterone levels. Metabolism 1990;39:897-901.

281. Mårin P, Lönn L, Andersson B, Oden B, Olbe L, Bengtsson B-À, Björntorp P: Assimilation of triglycerides in subcutaneous and intraabdominsl adipose tissues in vivo in men: effects of testosterone. Journal of Clinical Endocrinology and Metabolism 1996;81:1018-1022.

282. Laaksonen DE, Niskanen L, Punnonen K, Nyyssonen K, Tuomainen TP, Valkonen VP, Salonen R, Salonen JT: Testosterone and sex hormone-binding globulin predict the metabolic syndrome and diabetes in middle-aged men. Diabetes Care 2004;27:1036-1041.

283. Elbers JMH, Asscheman H, Seidell JC, Megens JAJ, Gooren LJG: Long-Term Testosterone Administration Increases Visceral Fat in Female to Male Transsexuals. Journal of Clinical Endocrinology and Metabolism 1997;82:2045-2047.

284. Draper N, Walker EA, Bujalska IJ, Tomlinson JW, Chalder SM, Arlt W, Lavery GG, Bodendo O, Ray DW, Laing I, Malunowicz E, White PC, Hewison M, Mason PJ, Connell JM, Shackleton CHL, Stewart PM: Mutations in the genes encoding 11β–hydroxysteroid dehydrogenase type 1 and hexose-6-phosphate dehydrogenase interact to casue cortisone reductase deficiency. Nature Genetics 2003;34:434-439.

285. Garaulet M, Perex-Llamas F, Baraza JC, Garcia-Prieto MD, Fardy PS, Tebar FJ, Zamora S: Body fat distribution inpre- and post-menopausal women: metabolic and anthropometric variables. Journal of Nutrition, Health & Aging 2002;6:123-126.

286. Leenen R, van der Kooy K, Seidell JC, Deurenberg P, Koppeschaar HPF: Visceral Fat Accumulation in Relation to Sex Hormones in Obese Men and Women Undergoing Weight Loss Therapy. Journal of Clinical Endocrinology and Metabolism 1994;78:1515-1520.

287. Sumino H, Ichikawa S, Yoshida A, Murakami M, Kanda T, Mizunuma H, Sakami T, Kurabayashi M: Effects of hormone replacement therapy on weight, abdominal fat distribution, and lipid levels in Japanese postmenopausal women. International Journal of Obesity and Related Metabolic Disorders 2003;27:1044-1051.

288. Rossouw JE, Anderson GL, Prentice RL, LaCroix AZ, Kooperberg C, Stefanick ML, Jackson RD, Beresford SA, Howard BV, Johnson KC, Kotchen JM, Ockene J: Risks and Benefits of Estrogen plus Progestin in Healthy Postmenopausal Women. JAMA 2002;288:321-333.

289. Cigolini M, Targher G, Bergamo Andreis IA, Tonoli M, Filippi F, Muggeo M, De Sandre G: Moderate alcohol consumption and its relation to visceral fat and plasma androgens in healthy women. International Journal of Obesity and Related Metabolic Disorders 1996;20:206-212.

290. Pasco A, Lemieux S, Lemieux I, Prud'homme D, Tremblay A, Bouchard C, Nadeau A, Couillard C, Tchernof A, Bergeron J, Després J-P: Age-Related Increase in Visceral Adipose Tissue and Body Fat and the Metabolic Risk Profile of Premenopausal Women. Diabetes Care 1999;22:1471-1478.

291. Clasey JL, Weltman A, Patrie J, Weltman JY, Pezzoli S, Bouchard C, Thorner MO, Hartman ML: Abdominal Visceral Fat and Fasting Insulin Are Important Predictors of 24-Hour GH Release Independent of Age, Gender, and Other Physiological Factors. Journal of Clinical Endocrinology and Metabolism 2001;86:3845-3852.

292. Isidori AM, Strollo F, Morè M, Caprio M, Aversa A, Moretti C, Frajese G, Riondino G, Fabbri A: Leptin and Aging: Correlation with Endocrine Changes in Male and Female Healthy Adult Populations of Different Body Weights. Journal of Clinical Endocrinology and Metabolism 2000;85:1954-1962.

293. Vogelzangs N, Kritchevsky SB, Beekman AT, Newman AB, Satterfield S, Simonsick EM, Yaffe K, Harris TB, Penninx BW: Depressive symptoms and change in abdominal obesity in older persons. Archives of General Psychiatry 2008;65:1386-1393.

294. Lonnqvist F, Nyberg B, Wahrenberg H, Arner P: Catecholamine-induced lipolysis in adipose tissue of the elderly. Journal of Clinical Investigation 1990;85:1614-1621.

295. Short KR, Vittone JL, Bigelow ML, Proctor DN, Sreekumaran Nair K: Age and aerobic exercise training effects on whole body and muscle protein metabolism. American Journal of Physiology 2004;286:E92-E101.

296. Schwartz RS, Jaeger LF, Veith RC: The thermic effect of feeding in older men: the importance of the sympaqthetic nervous system. Metabolism 1990;39:733-737.

297. Kerckhoffs DAJM, Blaak EE, Van Baak MA, Saris WHM: Effect of aging on $\square$–adrenergically mediated thermogenesis in men. American Journal of Physiology 1998;274:E1075-E1079.

298. Sial S, Coggan AR, Carroll R, Goodwin J, Klein S: Fat and carbohydrate metabolism during exercise in elderly and young subjects. American Journal of Physiology 1996;271:E983-E989.

299. Blaak EE, Van Baak MA, Saris WHM: $\square$-Adrenergically Stimulated Fat Oxidation is Diminished in Middle-Aged Compared to Young Subjects. Journal of Clinical Endocrinology and Metabolism 1999;84:3764-3769.

300. Ferraro R, Lillioja S, Fontvieille A-M, Rising R, Bogardus C, Ravussin E: Lower Sedentary Metabolic Rates in Women Comkpared with Men. Journal of Clinical Investigation 1992;90:780-784.

301. Ibáñez L, Lopez-Bermejo A, Suárez L, Marcos MV, Diaz M, Zegher Fd: Visceral Adiposity without Overweight in Children Born Small for Gestational Age. Journal of Clinical Endocrinology and Metabolism 2008;93:2079-2083.

302. Schwartz MB, Chambliss HO, Brownell KD, Blair SN, Billington C: Weight Bias among Health Professionals Specializing in Obesity. Obesity Research 2003;11:1033-1039.

303. Puhl R, Brownell KD: Bias, discrimination, and obesity. Obesity Research 2001;9:788-805.

304. Sonne-Holm S, Sorenson TI: Prospective study of attainment of social class of severely obese subjects in relation to parental social class, intelligence, and education. British Medical Journal 1986;292:586-589.

305. Wadden TA, Stunkard AJ: Social and Psychological Consequences of Obesity. Annals of Internal Medicine 1985;103:1062-1067.

306. Finkelstein, E. A., Fiebelkorn, I. C., and Wang, G. State-Level Estimates of Annual Medical Expenditures Attributable to Obesity. Obesity Research 12, 18-24. 2004.

307. Wang, G. and Dietz, W. H. Economic Burden of Obesity in Youths Aged 6 to 17 Years:1979-1999. Pediatrics 109, E81-1. 2002.

308. Daviglus, M. L., Liu, K., Yan, L. L., Pirzada, A., Manheim, L., Manning, W., Garside, D. B., Wang, R., Dyer, A. R, Greenland, P., and Stamler, J. Relation of Body Mass Index in Young Adulthood and Middle Age to Medicare Expenditures in Older Age. JAMA 292, 2743-2749. 2004.

309. Raebel, M. A., Malone, D. C., Conner, D. A., Xu, S., Porter, J. A., and Lanty, F. A. Health Services Use and Health Care Costs of Obese and Nonobese Individuals. Archives of Internal Medicine 164, 2135-2140. 2004.

310. Deurenberg P, Yap M, van Staveren WA: Body mass index and percent body fat: a meta analysis among different ethnic groups. International Journal of Obesity and Related Metabolic Disorders 1998;22:1164-1171.

311. Fernandez JE, Heo M, Heymsfield S, Pierson JrRN, Pi-Sunyer FX, Wang Z, Wang J, Hayes M, Allison DB, Gallagher D: Is percentage body aft differentially related to body mass index din Hispanic Americans, African Americans, and European Americans. American Journal of Clinical Nutrition 2003;77:71-75.

312. Clasey JL, Kanaley JA, Wideman L, Heymsfield S, Teates CD, Gutgesell ME, Thorner MO, Hartman ML, Weltman A: Validity of methods of body composition assessment in younger and older men and women. Journal of Applied Physiology 2000;89:2518-2520.

313. Sun SS, Chumlea WC, Heymsfield SB, Lukaski HC, Schoeller D, Friedl K, Kuczmarski RJ, Flegal KM, Johnson CL, Hubbard VS: Development of bioelectrical impedance analysis prediction equations for body composition with the use of a multicomponent model for use in epidemiologic surveys. American Journal of Clinical Nutrition 2003;77:331-340.

314. National Heart,Lung and Blood Institute Obesity Education Initiative. Clinical Guidelines on the Identification, Evaluation, and Treatment of Overweight and Obesity in Adults. 98-4083, 1-228. 1998. National Heart, Lung, and Blood Institute.

315. Van Itallie TB: Health implications of overweight and obesity in the United States. Annals of Internal Medicine 1985;6:983-988.

316. Manson JE, Stampter MJ, Hennekens CH, Willett WC: Body weight and longevity. A Reassessment. JAMA 1987;257:353-358.

317. Troiano RP, Frongillo EAJr, Sobal J, Levitsky DA: The relationship between body weight and mortality: a quantitative analysis of combined information from existing studies. International Journal of Obesity and Related Metabolic Disorders 1996;20:63-75.

318. Flegal KM, Carroll MD, Kuczmarski RJ, Johnson CL: Overweight and obesity in the United States: prevalence and trends, 1960-1994. International Journal of Obesity 1998;22:39-47.

319. Dublin LI: The influence of weight on certain causes of death. Human Biology 1930;2:159-184.

320. Peeters A, Barendregt JJ, Willekens F, Mackenbach JP, Mamun AA, Bonneux L: Obesity in Adulthood and Its Consequences for Life Expectancy: A Life-Table Analysis. Annals of Internal Medicine 2003;138:24-32.

321. Lee IM, Manson JE, Hennekens CH, Paffenbarger RSJr: Body weight and mortality. A 27-year follow-up of middle-aged men. JAMA 1993;270:2823-2828.

322. Meyer HE, Søgaard AJ, Tverdal A, Selmer RM: Body mass index and mortality: the influence of physical activity and smoking. Medicine and Science in Sports and Exercise 2002;34:1065-1070.

323. Sempos CT, Durazo-Arvizu R, McGee DL, Cooper RS, Prewitt TE: The influence of cigarette smoking on the association between body weight and mortality. The Framingham Study revisited. Annals of Epidemiology 2004;8:289-300.

324. Strawbridge WJ, Wallhagen MI, Shema SJ: New NHLBI Clinical Guidelines for Obesity and Overweight: Will They Promote Health? American Journal of Public Health 2000;90:340-343.

325. Visscher TL, Seidell JC, Menotti A, Blackburn H, Nissinen A, Freskens EJ, Kromhout D: Underweight and overweight in relation to mortality among men aged 40-59 and 50-69 years: the Seven Countries Study. American Journal of Epidemiology 2000;151:660-666.

326. Calle EE, Thun MJ, Petrelli JM, Rodriguez C, Heath CWJr: Body-mass index and mortality in a prospective cohort of U.S. adults. New England Journal of Medicine 1999;341:1097-1105.

327. Stevens J, Cai J, Pamuk ER, Williamson DF, Thun MJ, Wood JL: The effect of age on the association between body-mass index and mortality. New England Journal of Medicine 1998;338:1-7.

328. Flicker L, McCaul KA, Hankey GJ, Jamrozik K, Brown WJ, Byles JE, Almeida OP: Body Mass Index and Survival in Men and Women Aged 70 to 75. Journal of American Geriatric Society 2010;58:234-241.

329. Heiat A, Vaccarino V, Krumholz HM: An Evidence-Based Assessment of Federal Guidelines for Overweight and Obesity as They Apply to Elderly Persons. Archives of Internal Medicine 2001;161:1194-1203.

330. Franks PW, Hanson RL, Knowler WC, Sievers ML, Bennett PH, Looker HC: Childhood Obesity, Other Cardiovascular Risk Factors,. and Premature Death. New England Journal of Medicine 2010;362:485-493.

331. Rosenberg L, Czene K, Hall P: Obesity and poor breast cancer prognosis: an illusion because of hormone replacement therapy? British Journal of Cancer 2009;100:1486-1491.

332. Stevens J, Juhaeri, Cai J, Jones DW: The effect of decision rules on the choice of a body mass index cutoff for obesity: examples from Africqan-American and white women. American Journal of Clinical Nutrition 2002;75:986-992.

333. Lee CD, Blair SN, Jackson AS: Cardiorespiratory fitness, body composition, and all-cause and cardiovascular disease mortality in men. American Journal of Clinical Nutrition 1999;69:373-380.

334. Wei M, Kampert JB, Barlow CE, Nichaman MZ, Gibbons LW, Paffenbarger RS Jr, Blair SN: Relationship Between Low Cardiorespiratory Fitness and Mortality in Normal-weight, Overweight, and Obese Men. JAMA 1999;282:1547-1553.

335. Stevens J, Cai J, Evenson KR, Thomas R: Fitness and Fatness as Predictors of Mortality from All Causes and from Cardiovascular Disease in Men and Women in the Lipid Research Clinics Study. American Journal of Epidemiology 2002;156:832-841.

336. Sui X, LaMonte MJ, Laditka JN, Hardin JW, Chase N, Hooker SP, Blair SN: Cardiorespiratory Fitness and Adiposity as Mortality Predictors in Older Adults. JAMA 2007;298:2507-2516.

337. Flegal KM, Graubard BI, Williamson DF, Gail MH: Excess Deaths Associated With Underweight, Overweight, and Obesity. JAMA 2005;293:1861-1867.

338. Mokdad AH, Marks JS, Stroup DF, Gerberding JL: Actual Cause of Death in the United States, 2000. JAMA 2005;291:1238-1245.

339. Katzmarzyk PT, Craig CL, Bouchard C: Original Article Underweight, overweight and obesity: relationships with mortality in the 13-year followup of the Canadian Fitness Survey. Journal of Clinical Epidemiology 2001;54:916-920.

340. Gregg EW, Cheng YJ, Cadwell BL, Imperatore G, Williams DE, Flegal KM, Narayan KMV, Williamson DF: Secular Trends in Cardiovascular Disease Risk Factors According to Body Mass Index in US Adults. JAMA 2005;293:1868-1874.

341. Haapanen-Niemi N, Miilunpalo S, Vuori I, Oja P, Malmberg J: Body mass index, physical inactivity and low level of physical fitness as determinants of all cause and cardiovascular disease mortality - 16 y follow-up of middle-aged and elderly men and women. International Journal of Obesity 2000;24:1465-1474.

342. Secareccia F, Lanti M, Menotti A, Scanga M: Role of body mass index in the prediction of all cause mortality in over 62,000 men and women. The Italian RIFLE Pooling Project. Journal of Epidemiology and Community Health 1998;52:20-26.

343. Bender R, Trautner C, Spraul M, Berger M: Assessment of excess mortality in obesity. American Journal of Epidemiology 1998;147:42-48.

344. Must A, Spadano J, Coakley EH, Field AE, Colditz G, Dietz WH: The Disease Burden Associated with Overweight and Obesity. JAMA 1999;282:1523-1529.

345. McTigue KM, Garrett JM, Popkin BM: The Natural History of the Development of Obesity in a Cohort of Young U.S. Adults between 1981 and 1998. Annals of Internal Medicine 2002;136:857-864.

346. Thorpe, K. E., Florence, C. S., Howard, D. H., and Joski, P. The Rising Prevalence Of Treated Disease: Effects On Private Health Insurance Spending. Health Affairs . 2005.

347. Adams KF, Schatzkin A, Harris TB, Kipnis V, Mouw T, Ballard-Barbash R, Hollenbeck A, Leitzman MF: Overweight, Obesity, and Mortality in a Large Prospective Cohort of Persons 50 to 71 Years Old. New England Journal of Medicine 2006;355:763-778.

348. Jee SH, Sull JW, Park J, Lee S-Y, Ohrr H, Guallar E, Samet JM: Body-Mass Index and Mortality in Korean Men and Women. New England Journal of Medicine 2006;355:779-787.

349. Bigaard J, Tjønneland A, Thomsen BL, Overvad K, Heitman BL, Sørensen TIA: Waist Circumference, BMI, Smoking, and Mortality in Middle-aged Men and Women. Obesity Research 2003;11:895-903.

350. Yusuf S, Hawken S, Ounpuu S, Bautista L, Franzosi MG, Commerford P, Lang CC, Rumbold Z, Onen CL, Lisheng L, Tanomsup S, Wangai SJr, Razak F, Sharma AM, Anand SS, INTERHEART Study Investigators: Obesity and the risk of myocardial infarction in 27,000 participants from 52 countries: a case-control study. Lancet 2005;366:1640-1649.

351. Mark DH: Deaths Attributable to Obesity. JAMA 2005;293:1918-1919.

352. Calle EE, Rodriguez C, Walker-Thurmond K, Thun MJ: Overweight, and mortality from cancer in a prospectively studied cohort of U.S. adults. New England Journal of Medicine 2003;348:1625-1638.

353. Key TJ, Appleby PN, Reeves GK, Roddam A, Dorgan JF, Longcope C, Stanczyk FZ, Stephenson HEJr, Falk RT, Miller R, Schatzkin A, Allen DS, Fentiman IS, Key TJ, Wang DY, Dowsett M, Thomas HV, Hankinson SE, Toniolo P, Akhmedkhanov A, Koenig K, Shore RE, Zeleniuch-Jaquotte A, Berrino F, Muti P, Micheli A, Krogh V, Sieri S, Pala V, Venturelli E, Secreto G, Barret-Connor E, Laughlin GA, Kabuto M, Akiba S, Stevens RG, Neriish K, Land CE, Cauley JA, Kuller LH, Cummings SR, Helzlsouer KJ, Alberg AJ, Bush TL, Comstock GW, Gordon GB, Miller SR, Longcope C: Body mass index, serum sex hormones, and breast cancer risk in postmenopausal women. Journal of National Cancer Institute 2003;95:1218-1226.

354. Rodriguez C, Patel AV, Calle EE, Jacobs EJ, Chao A, Thun MJ: Body Mass Index, Height, and Prostate Cancer Mortality in Two Large Cohorts of Adult Men in the United States. Cancer Epidemiology, Biomarkers & Prevention 2001;10:345-353.

355. Moore LL, Bradlee ML, Splansky GL, Proctor MH, Ellison RC, Kreger IBE: BMI and waist circumference as predictors of lifetime colon cancer risk in Framingham Study adults. International Journal of Obesity and Related Metabolic Disorders 2004;28:559-567.

356. Meyerhardt JA, Catalano PJ, Heller DG, Mayer RJ, Benson IAB, Macdonald JS, Fuchs CS: Influence of body mass index on outcomes and treatment-related toxicity in patients with colon carcinoma. Cancer 2003;98:484-495.

357. Murphy TK, Calle EE, Rodriguez C, Khan HS, Thun MJ: Body mass index and colon cancer mortality in a large prospective study. American Journal of Epidemiology 2000;152:847-854.

358. Tavani A, La Vecchia C: Epidemiology of renal-cell carcinoma. Journal of Nephrology 1997;10:93-106.

359. Furberg A-S, Thune I: Metabolic abnormalities (hypertension, hyperglycemia and overweight), lifestyle (high energy intake and physical inactivity) and endometrial cancer risk in a Norwegian cohort. International Journal of Cancer 2003;104:669-678.

360. Maclure KM, Hayes KC, Colditz GA, Stampfer MJ, Speizer FE, Willett WC: Weight, diet, and the risk of symptomatic gallstones in middle-aged women. New England Journal of Medicine 1989;321:563-569.

361. Jensen DM, Damm P, Serensen B, Mølsted-Pedersen L, Westergaard JG, Ovesen P, Beck-Nielsen H: Pregnancy outcome and prepregnancy body mass index in 2459 glucose-tolerant Danish women. American Journal of Obstetrics and Gynecology 2003;189:239-244.

362. Rosengren, A., Skoog, I., Gustafson, D., and Wilhelmsen, L. Body Mass Index, Other Cardiovascular Risk Factors and Hospitalization for Dementia. Archives of Internal Medicine 165, 321-326. 2005.

363. Gustafson D, Rothenberg E, Blennow K, Steen B, Skoog I: An 18-year follow-up of overweight and risk of Alzheimer disease. Archives of Internal Medicine 2003;163:1524-1528.

364. Whitmer, R. A., Gunderson, E. P., Barrett-Connor, E., Queensberry, C. P., and Yaffe, K. Obesity in middle age and future risk of dementia: a 27 year longitudinal population based study. British Medical Journal . 2005. Ref Type: Electronic Citation

365. Thomas EJ, Goldman L, Mangione CM, Marcantonio ER, Cook EF, Ludwig L, Sugarbaker D, Poss R, Donaldson M, Lee TH: Body Mass Index as a Correlate of Postoperative Complications and Resource Utilization. American Journal of Medicine 1997;103:277-283.

366. Cooper C, Snow S, McAlindon TE, Kellingray S, Stuart B, Coggon D, Dieppe PA: Risk factors for the incidence and progression of radiographic knee osteoarthritis. Arthritis and Rheumatism 2000;43:995-1000.

367. Wilson LJ, Hirschowitz BI: Association of obesity with hiatal hernia and esophagitis. American Journal of Gastroenterology 1999;94:2840-2844.

368. Sharp JT, Henry JP, Sweany SK, Meadows WR, Pietras RJ: The Total Work of Breathing in Normal and Obese Men. Journal of Clinical Investigation 1964;43:728-739.

369. Young T, Dempsey J, Skatrud J, Weber S, Badr S: The Occurrence of Sleep-Disordered Breathing among Middle-Aged Adults. New England Journal of Medicine 1993;328:1230-1235.

370. Dalloso HM, McGrother CW, Mathews RJ, Donaldson MM: The association of diet and other lifestyle factors with overactive bladder and stress incontinence: a longitudinal study in women. British Journal of Urology International 2003;92:69-77.

371. Moore LL, Singer MR, Bradlee ML, Rothman KJ, Milunsky A: A prospective study of the risk of congenital defects associated with maternal obesity and diabetes mellitus. Epidemiology 2000;11:689-694.

372. Kenchaiah S, Evans JC, Levy D, Wilson PWF, Benjamin EJ, Larson MG, Kannel WB, Vasan RS: Obesity and the Risk of Heart Failure. New England Journal of Medicine 2002;347:305-313.

373. Elmore JG, Carney PA, Abraham LA, Barlow WE, Egger JR, Fosse JS, Cutter GR, Hendrick RE, D'Orsi CJ, Paliwal P, Taplin SH: The association between obesity and screening mammography accuracy. Archives of Internal Medicine 2004;164:1140-1147.

374. Choi HK, Atkinson K, Karlson EW, Curhan G: Obesity, Weight Change, Hypertension, Diuretic Use, and Risk of Gout in Men. Archives of Internal Medicine 2005;165:742-748.

375. Jood K, Jern C, Wilhelmsen L, Rosengren A: Body mass index in mid-life is associated with a first stroke in men: a prospective population study over 28 years. Stroke 2004;35:2764-2769.

376. Taylor EN, Stampfer MJ, Curhan GC: Obesity, Weight Gain, and the Risk of Kidney Stones. JAMA 2006;293:455-462.

377. Ruhl CE, Everhart JE: Determinants of the association of overweight with elevated serum alanine aminotransferase activity in the United States. Gastroenterology 2003;124:248-250.

378. National Cholesterol Education Program Expert Panel on Detection, Evaluation, and Treatment of High Blood Cholesterol in Adults (Adult Treatment Panel III). Third Report of the National Cholesterol Education Expert Panel on Detection, Evaluation, and Treatment of High Blood Cholesterol in Adults (Adult Treatment Panel III). 01-3670, 1-27. 2001. National Institutes of Health.

379. Alberti KGMM, Eckel RH, Grundy SM, Zimmet PZ, Cleeman JI, Donato KA, Fruchart J-C, James PT, Loria CM, Smith JrSC: Harmonizing the Metabolic Syndrome. A Joint Interim Statement of the Intrernational Diabetes Federation Task Force on Epidemiology and Prevention; American Heart Association; World Heart Federation; International Atherosclerosis Society; and International Association for the Study of Obesity. Circulation 2009;120:1640-1645.

380. Park YW, Zhu S, Palaniappan L, Heshka S, Carnethon MR, Heymsfield SB: The Metabolic Syndrome. Archives of Internal Medicine 2003;163:427-436.

381. Ford ES, Giles WH, Dietz WH: Prevalence of the Metabolic Syndrome Among US Adults. JAMA 2002;287:356-359.

382. Weiss R, Dziura J, Burgert TS, Tamborlane WV, Taksali SE, Yeckel CW, Allen K, Lopes M, Savoye M, Morrison J, Sherwin RS, Caprio S: Obesity and the Metabolic Syndrome in Children and Adolescents. New England Journal of Medicine 2004;350:2362-2374.

383. Gorter PM, Olijhoek JB, van der Graaf Y, Algra A, Rabelink TJ, Visseren FLJ: Prevalence of the metabolic syndrome in patients with coronary heart disease, peripheral arterial disease or abdominal aortic aneurysm. Atherosclerosis 2004;173:361-367.

384. Hu G, Qiao Q, Tuomilehto J, Balkau B, Borch-Johnsen K, Pyorala K: Prevalence of the metabolic syndrome and its relation to all-cause and cardiovascular mortality in nondiabetic European men and women. Archives of Internal Medicine 2004;164:1066-1076.

385. Katzmarzyk PT, Church TS, Blair SN: Cardiorespiratory fitness attenuates the effects of the metabolic syndrome on all-cause and cardiovascular disease mortality in men. Archives of Internal Medicine 2004;164:1092-1097.

386. Kip KE, Marroquin OC, Kelley DE, Johnson BD, Kelsey SF, Shaw LJ, Rogers WJ, Reis SE: Clinical Importance of Obesity Versus the Metabolic Syndrome in Cardiovascular Risk in Women. Circulation 2004;109:706-713.

387. Marroquin OC, Kip KE, Kelley DE, Johnson BD, Shaw LJ, Bairey Merz CN, Sharaf BL, Pepine CJ, Sopko G, Reis SE, Women's Ischemia Syndrome Evaluation Investigators: Metabolic syndrome modifies the cardiovascular risk associated with angiographic coronary artery disease in women: a report from the Women's Ischemia Syndrome Evaluation. Circulation 2004;109:714-721.

388. Katzmarzyk PT, Church TS, Janssen I, Ross R, Blair SN: Metabolic syndrome, obesity, and mortality: impact of cardiorespiratory fitness. Diabetes Care 2005;28:391-397.

389. Cornier AS, Tate CW, Grunwald GK, Bessesen DH: Relationship between waist circumference, body mass index, and medical care costs. Obesity Research 2002;10:1167-1172.

390. Wilson PW, Kannel WB, Silberschatz H, D'Agostino RB: Clustering of metabolic factors and coronary heart disease. Archives of Internal Medicine 1999;159:1104-1109.

391. Kahn R, Buse J, Ferrannini E, Stern M: The Metabolic Syndrome: Time for a Critical Appraisal. Diabetes Care 2005;28:2289-2304.

392. Karelis AD, St-Pierre DH, Conus F, Rabasa-Lhoret R, Poehlman ET: Metabolic and Body Composition Factors in Subgroups of Obesity: What Do We Know? Journal of Clinical Endocrinology and Metabolism 2004;89:2569-2575.

393. Goodpaster BH, Krishnaswami S, Harris TB, Katsiaris A, Kritchevsky SB, Simonsick EM, Nevitt M, Holvoet P, Newman AB: Obesity, Regional Body Fat Distribution, and the Metabolic Syndrome in Older Men and Women. Archives of Internal Medicine 2005;165:777-783.

394. Sims EA: Are there persons who are obese, but metabolically healthy? Metabolism 2001;50:1499-1504.

395. Atkinson RL, Durandhar NV, Allison DB, Bowen RL, Israel BA, Albu JB, Augstus AS: Human adenovirus-36 is associated with increased body weight and paradoxical reduction of serum lipids. International Journal of Obesity 2005;29:281-286.

396. Lean MEJ, Han TS, Morrison CE: Waist circumference as a measure for indicating need for weight management. British Medical Journal 1995;311:158-161.

397. Zhu S, Wang Z, Heshka S, Heo M, Faith MS, Heymsfield SB: Waist circumference and obesity-associated risk factors among whites in the third National Health and Nutrition Examination Survey: clinical action thresholds. American Journal of Clinical Nutrition 2002;76:743-749.

398. Janssen I, Katzmarzyk PT, Ross R: Body Mass Index, Waist Circumference, and Health Risk. Archives of Internal Medicine 2002;162:2074-2079.

399. Okosun IS, Boltri JM, Eriksen MP, Hepburn VA: Trends in abdominal obesity in young people: United States 1988-2002. Ethnicity & Disease 2006;16:338-344.

400. Brambilla P, Bedogni G, Moreno LA, Goran MI, Gutin B, Fox KR, Peters DM, Barbeau P, De Simone M, Pietrobelli A: Crossvalidation of anthropometry against magnetic resonance imaging for the assessment of visceral and adipose tissue in children. International Journal of Obesity 2006;30:23-30.

401. Holvoet P, Kritchevsky SB, Tracy RP, Mertens A, Rubin SM, Butler J, Goodpaster B, Harris TB: The metabolic syndrome, circulating oxidized LDL, and risk of myocardial infarction in well-functioning elderly people in the health, aging, and body composition cohort. Diabetes 2004;53:1068-1073.

402. Sattar N, Gaw A, Scherbakova O, Ford I, O'Reilly DStJ, Haffner SM, Isles C, Macfarlane PW, Packard CJ, Cobbe SM, Shepherd J: Metabolic Syndrome With and Without C-Reactive Protein as a Predictor of Coronary Heart Disease and Diabetes in the West of Scotland Coronary Prevention Study. Circulation 2003;108:414-419.

403. Rutter MK, Meigs JB, Sullivan LM, D'Agostino RBSr, Wilson PW: C-reactive protein, the metabolic syndrome, and prediction of cardiovascular events in the Framingham Offspring Study. Circulation 2004;110:380-385.

404. Cereda E, Sansone V, Meola G, Malavazos AE: Increased visceral adipose tissue rather than BMI as a risk factor for dementia. Age and Ageing 2007;36:488-491.

405. Elias MF, Elias PK, Sullivan LM, Wolf PA, D'Agostino RB: Obesity, diabetes and cognitive deficit: The Framingham Heart Study. Neurobiology of Aging 2005;21:11-16.

406. Raji, C. A., Ho, A. J., Parikshak, N. N., Becker, J. T., Lopez, O. L., Kuller, L. H., Hua, X., Leow, A. D., Toga, A. W., and Thompson, P. M. Brain Structure and Obesity. 2009.

407. Kushner, R. F. Evaluating Your Patients for Overweight and Obesity. 2, 1-21. 2003. Chicago, Ill., American Medical Association. Roadmaps for Clinical Practice: Case Studies in Disease Prevention and Health Promotion-Assessment and Management of Adult Obesity: A Primer for Physicians.

408. Wajchenberg BL: Subcutaneous and Visceral Adipose Tissue: Their Relation to the Metabolic Syndrome. Endocrine Reviews 2000;21:697-738.

409. Nicklas BJ, Berman DM, Phennix BWJH, Lynch NA, Ryan AS, Dennis KE: Visceral Adipose Tissue Cutoffs Associated with Metabolic Risk Factor for Coronary Heart Disease in Women. Diabetes Care 2003;26:1413-1420.

410. Rossner S, Bo WJ, Hiltbrandt E, Hinson W, Karstaedt N, Santago P, Sobol WT, Crouse JR: Adipose tissue determinations in cadavers-a comparison between cross-sectional planimetry and computed tomography. International Journal of Obesity 1990;14:893-902.

411. Greenfield JR, Samaras K, Chisholm DJ, Campbell LV: Regional Intra-Subject Variability in Abdominsl Adiposity Limits Usefulness of Computed Tomography. Obesity Research 2002;10:260-265.

412. Kvist H, Sjöström L, Tylén U: Adipose tissue volume determinations in women by computed tomography: technical considerations. International Journal of Obesity 1986;10:53-67.

413. Sumner AE, Farmer NM, Tulloch-Reid MK, Sebring NG, Yanovski JA, Reynolds JC, Boston RC, Premkumar A: Sex differences in visceral adipose tissue volume among African-Americans. American Journal of Clinical Nutrition 2002;76:975-979.

414. Thomas EL, Saeed N, Hajnal JV, Brynes A, Goldstone AP, Frost G, Dell JD: Magnetic resonance imaging of total body fat. Journal of Applied Physiology 1998;85:1778-1785.

415. Fowler PA, Fuller MF, Glasbey CA, Cameron GG, Foster MA: Validation of the in vivo measurement of adipose tissue by magnetic resonance imaging of lean and obese pigs. American Journal of Clinical Nutrition 1992;56:7-13.

416. Abate N, Burns D, Peshock RM, Garg A, Grundy SM: Estimation of adipose tissue mass by magnetic resonance imaging: validation against dissection in human cadavers. Journal of Lipid Research 1994;35:1490-1496.

417. Anderson PJ, Chan JC, Chan YL, Tomlinson B, Young RP, Lee ZS, Lee KK, Metreweli C, Cockram CS, Critchley JA: Visceral fat and cardiovascular risk factors in Chinese NIDDM patients. Diabetes Care 1997;20:1854-1858.

418. Stolk RP, Wink O, Zelissen PM, Meijer R, van Gils AP, Grobbee DE: Validity and reproducibility of ultrasonography for the measurement of intra-abdominal adipose tissue. International Journal of Obesity and Related Metabolic Disorders 2001;25:1346-1351.

419. Stolk RP, Meijer R, Mali WPTM, Grobbee DE, van der Graaf Y: Ultrasound measurements of intraabdominal fat estimate the metabolic syndrome better than do measurements of waist circumference. American Journal of Clinical Nutrition 2003;77:857-860.

420. Martin AD, Daniel MZ, Drinkwater DT, Clarys JP: Adipose tissue density, estimated adipose lipid fraction and whole body adiposity in male cadavers. International Journal of Obesity 1994;18:79-83.

421. Bays H, Mandarino L, DeFronzo RA: Role of the Adipocyte. Free Fatty Acids, and Ectopic Fat in Pathogenesis of Type 2 Diabetes Mellitus: Peroxisomal Proliferator-Activated Receptor Agonists Provide a Rational Therapeutic Approach. Journal of Clinical Endocrinology and Metabolism 2004;89:463-478.

422. Garg A: Lipodystrophies. American Journal of Medicine 2000;108:143-152.

423. Marceau P, Biron S, Hould F-S, Marceau S, Simard S, Thung S, Kral JG: Liver Pathology and the Metabolic Syndrome X Severe Obesity. Journal of Clinical Endocrinology and Metabolism 1999;84:1513-1517.

424. Marchesini G, Brizi M, Bianchi G, Tomassetti S, Bugianesi E, Lenzi M, McCullough AJ, Natale S, Fiorlani G, Melchionda N: Nonalcoholic Fatty Liver Disease A Feature of the Metabolic Syndrome. Diabetes 2001;50:1844-1850.

425. Wang C-P, Chung F-M, Shin S-J, Lee Y-J: Congenitall and Environmental Factors Associated with Adipocyte Dysregulation as Defects of Insulin Resistance. Review of Diabetic Studies 2007;4:77-84.

426. Rasouli N, Kern PA: Adipocytokines and the Metabolic Complications of Obesity. Journal of Clinical Endocrinology and Metabolism 2008;93:S64-S73.

427. Tilg H, Moschen AR: Role of adiponectin and PBEF/visfatin as regulators of inflammation: involvement in obesity-associated diseases. Clinical Science 2008;114:275-288.

428. Meshkani, R. and Adeli, K. Hepatic insulin resistance, metabolic syndrome and cardiovascular disease. Clinical Biochemistry . 2009.

429. Mohan V, Deepa R, Pradeepa R, Vimalesdwaran KS, Mohan A, Velmurugan K, Radha V: Association of low adiponectin levels with the metabolic syndrome - the Chennai Rural Epidemiology Study (CURES-4). Metabolism 2005;54:476-481.

430. Lin E, Phillips LS, Ziegler TR, Schmotzer B, Kongjun W, Gu LH, Khaitan L, Lynch SA, Torres WE, Smith CD, Gletsu-Miller N: Increases in Adiponectin Prerdict Improved Liver, but Not Peripheral, Insulin Sensitiivity in Severely Obese Women During Weight Loss. Diabetes 2007;56:735-742.

431. Madsen EL, Rissanen A, Bruun JM, Skogstrand K, Tonstad S, Hougaard DM, Richelsen B: Weight loss larger than 10% is needed for general improvement of leveld of circulating adiponectin and markers of inflammation in obese subjects: a 3-year weight loss study. European Journal of Endocrinology 2008;158:179-187.

432. Yamauchi T, Kamon J, Waki H, Terauchi Y, Kubota N, Hara K, Mori Y, Ide T, Murakami K, Tsuboyama-Kasaoka N, Ezaki O, Akanuma Y, Gavrilovna O, Vinson C, Reitman ML, Kagechika H, Shudo K, Yoda M, Nakano Y, Tobe K, Nagai R, Kimura S, Tomita M, Froguel P, Kadowaki T: The fat-derived hormone adiponectin reverses insulin resistance associated with both lipoatrophy and obesity. Nature Medicine 2001;7:941-946.

433. Li L, Yang G, Shi S, Yang M, Liu H, Boden G: The adipose triglyceride lipase, adiponectin and visfatin are down regulated by tumor necrosis factor-alpha (TNF-alpha) in vivo. Cytokine 2009;45:12-19.

434. Dandona P, Weinstock R, Thusu K, Abdel-Rahman E, Aljada A, Wadden T: Tumor Necrosis Factor-⊠ in Sera of Obese Patients: Fall with Weight Loss. Journal of Clinical Endocrinology and Metabolism 1998;83:2907-2910.

435. Kopp HP, Kopp CW, Festa A, Krzyzanowska K, Kriwanek S, Minar E, Roka R, Schernthaner G: Impact of Weight Loss on Inflammatory Proteins and Their Association With the Insulin Resistance Syndrome in Morbidly Obese Patients. Arteriosclerosis, Thrombosis, and Vascular Biology 2003;23:1042-1047.

436. Klein S, Fontana L, Young VL, Coggan AR, Kilo C, Patterson BW, Mohammed BS: Absence of an Effect of Liposuction on Insulin Action and Risk Factors for Coronary Heart Disease. New England Journal of Medicine 2004;350:2549-2557.

437. Bastard J-P, Maachi M, Lagathu C, Kim MJ, Caron M, Vidal H, Capeau J, Feve B: Recent advances in the relationship between obesity, inflammation, and insulin resistance. European Cytokine Network 2006;17:4-12.

438. Goldstein BJ, Scalia RG, Ma XL: Protective vascular and myocardial effects of adiponectin. Nature Clinical Practise and Cardiovascular Medicine 2009;6:27-35.

439. Ronti T, Lupatelli G, Mannarino E: The endocrine function of adipose tissue: an update. Clinical Endocrinology 2006;64:355-365.

440. Zhu W, Cheng KKY, Vanhoutte PM, Lam KSL, Xu A: Vascular effects of adiponectin: molecular mechanisms and potential therapeutic intervention. Clinical Science 2008;114:361-374.

441. Kadowaki T, Yamauchi T, Kubota N, Hara K, Ueki K, Tobe K: Adiponectin and adiponectin receptors in insulin resistance, diabetes and the metabolic syndrome. Journal of Clinical Investigation 2006;116:1784-1792.

442. Pischon T, Nörthling U, Boeing H: Obesity and cancer. Proceedings of the Nutrition Society 2008;67:128-145.

443. Goldstein DJ: Beneficial Health effects of modest weight loss. International Journal of Obesity 1992;16:397-415.

444. Moore LL, Visioni AJ, Qureshi MM, Bradlee ML, Ellison RC, D'Agostino R: Weight Loss in Overweight Adults and the long-term Risk of Hypertension. Archives of Internal Medicine 2005;165:1298-1303.

445. Hensrud DD, Weinsier RL, Darnell BE, Hunter GR: Relationship of co-morbidities of obesity to weight loss and four year weight maintenance/rebound. Obesity Research 1995;3:217S-222S.

446. Esposito K, Giugliano F, Di Palo C, Giugliano C, Marfella R, D'Andrea F, D'Armiento M, Gugliano D: Effect of lifestyle changes on erectile dysfunction in obese men: a randomized controlled trial. JAMA 2004;291:2978-2984.

447. Focht BC, Rejeski WJ, Ambrosius WT, Katula JA, Messier SP: Exercise, self-efficacy, and mobility performance in overweight and obese older adults with knee osteoarthritis. Arthritis and Rheumatism 2005;53:659-665.

448. Park HS, Lee K: Greater Beneficial effects of visceral fat reduction compared with subcutaneous fat reduction on parameters of the metabolic syndrome: a study of weight reduction programmes in subjects with visceral and subcutaneous obesity. Diabetic Medicine 2005;22:266-272.

449. Leenen R, van der Kooy K, Deurenberg P, Seidell JC, Weststrate JA, Schouten FJ, Hautvast JG: Visceral fat accumulation in obese subjects: relation to energy expenditure and response to weight loss. American Journal of Physiology 1992;263:E913-E919.

450. Williamson DF, Pamuk ER: The Association between Weight Loss and Increased Longevity. Annals of Internal Medicine 1993;119:731-736.

451. Andres R, Muller DC, Sorkin JD: Long-term effects of change in body weight weight on all-cause mortality. A review. Annals of Internal Medicine 1993;120 Supplement 3:80-82.

452. Droyvold WB, Lund Nilsen TI, Lydersen S, Midthjell K, Nilsson PM, Nilsson JA, Holmen J: Weight change and mortality: the Nord-Trondelag Health Study. Journal of Internal Medicine 2005;257:338-345.

453. Sorensen TI: Weight loss causes increased mortality: pros. Obesity Reviews 2005;4:1-2.

454. Sørensen TIA, Rissanen A, Korkeila M, Kaprio J: Intention to Lose Weight, Weight Changes, and 18-y Mortality in Overweight Individuals without Co-Morbidities. PLOS MEDICINE 2005;2:e171.

455. Wannamethee SG, Shaper AG, Walker M: Weight change, weight fluctuation, and mortality. Archives of Internal Medicine 2002;162:2575-2580.

456. Williamson DF, Pamuk E, Thun M, Flanders D, Byers T, Heath C: Prospective study of intentional weight loss and mortality in overweight white men aged 40-64 years. American Journal of Epidemiology 1999;149:491-503.

457. Yaari S, Goldbourt U: Voluntary and involuntary weight loss: associations with long term mortality in 9,228 middle-aged and elderly men. American Journal of Epidemiology 1998;148:546-555.

458. French SA, Folson AR, Jeffery RW, Williamson DF: Prospective study of intentionality of weight loss and mortality in older women: the Iowa Women's Health Study. American Journal of Epidemiology 1999;149:504-514.

459. Gregg EW, Gerzoft RB, Thompson TJ, Williamson DF: Intentional Weight Loss and Death in Overweight and Obese U.S. Adults 35 Years of Age and Older. Annals of Internal Medicine 2003;138:383-389.

460. Wannamethee SG, Shaper AG, Lennon L: Reasons for Intentional Weight Loss, Unintentional Weight Loss and Mortality in Older Men. Archives of Internal Medicine 2005;165:1035-1040.

461. Williamson DF, Pamuk E, Thun M, Flanders D, Byers T, Heath C: Prospective study of intentional weight loss and mortality in never-smoking overweight US white women aged 40-64 years. American Journal of Epidemiology 1995;141:1128-1141.

462. Williamson DF, Thompson TJ, Thun M, Flanders D, Pamuk E, Byers T: Intentional Weight Loss and Mortality Among Overweight Individuals with Diabetes. Diabetes Care 2000;23:1499-1504.

463. Coffey CS, Gadbury GL, Fontaine KR, Wang C, Weindruch R, Allison DB: The effects of intentional weight loss as a latent variable problem. Statistics in Medicine 2005;24:941-954.

464. Dyer AR, Stamler J, Greenland P: Associations of weight change and weight variability with cardiovascular and all-cause mortality in the Chicago Western Electric Company Study. American Journal of Epidemiology 2000;152:324-333.

465. Cornoni-Huntley JC, Harris TB, Everett DF, Albanes D, Micozzi MS, Miles TP, Eldman JJ: An overview of body weight of older persons, including the impact on mortality. The National Health and Nutrition Examination Survey I-Epidemiologic Follow-up Study. Journal of Clinical Epidemiology 1991;44:743-753.

466. Harris T, Cook EF, Garrison R, Higgins M, Kannel W, Goldman L: Body mass index and mortality among nonsmoking older persons. The Framingham Heart Study. JAMA 1988;259:1520-1524.

467. Losonczy KG, Harris TB, Cornoni-Huntley JC, Simonsick EM, Wallace RB, Cook NR, Ostfeld AM, Blazer DG: Does weight loss from middle age to old age explain the inverse weight mortality relation in old age? American Journal of Epidemiology 1995;141:312-321.

468. Oreopoulos A, Padwal R, Kalantar-Zadeh K, Fonarow GC, Norris CM, McAlister FA: Body mass index and m ortality in heart failure: a meta-analysis. American Heart Journal 2008;156:13-22.

469. Dagenais GR, Mann JF, Bosch J, Pogue J, Yusuf S: Prognostic impact of body weight and abdominal obesity in women and men with cardiovascular disease. American Heart Journal 2005;149:54-60.

470. Evangelista LS, Heber D, Bowerman S, Hamilton MA, Fonarow GC: Reduced body weight and adiposity with a high protein diet improves functional status, lipid profiles, glycemic control, and quality of life in patients with heart failure: a feasibility study. Journal of Cardiovascular Nursing 2009;24:207-215.

471. Strandberg, T. E., Strandberg, A. Y., Salomaa, V. V., Pitkälä, K. H., Tilvis, R. S., Sirola, J., and Mietten, T. A. Explaining the obesity paradox: cardiovascular risk, weight change, and mortality during long-term follow-up in men. European Heart Journal . 2009.

472. Colman RJ, Anderson RM, Johnson SC, Kastman EK, Kosmatka KJ, Beasley TM, Allison DB, Cruzen C, Simmons HA, Kemnitz JW, Weindruch R: Caloric Restriction Delays Disease Onset and Mortality in Rhesus Monkeys. Science 2009;325:201-204.

473. Fontana L, Meyer TE, Klein S, Holloszy JO: Long-term calorie restriction is highly effective in reducing the risk for atherosclerosis in humans. Proceedings of the National Academy of Science 2004;101:6659-6663.

474. Meyer TE, Kovács SJ, Ehsani AA, Klein S, Holloszy JO, Fontana L: Long-Term Caloric Restriction Ameliorates the Decline in Diastolic Function in Humans. Journal of the American College of Cardiology 2006;47:398-402.

475. Roth, G. S., Lane, M. A., Ingram, D. K., Mattison, J. A., Elahi, D., Tobin, J. D., Muller, D., and Metter, E. J. Biomarkers of Caloric Restriction May Predict Longevity in Humans. Science 297, 811. 2002.

476. Stunkard AJ, Rush J: Dieting and Depression Reexamined. Annals of Internal Medicine 1974;81:526-533.

477. Smith SR, de Jonge L, Pellymounter M, Nguyen T, Harris R, York D, Redmann S, Rood J, Bray GA: Peripheral Administration of Human Corticotropin-Releasing Hormone: A novel Method to Increase Energy Expenditure and Fat Oxidation in Man. Journal of Clinical Endocrinology and Metabolism 2001;86:1991-1998.

478. Task Force on DSM-IV: Diagnostic and Statistical Manual of Mental Disorders, ed Fourth. Washington, DC, American Psychiatric Association, 1994.

479. Patton GC, Johnson-Sabine E, Wood K, Mann AH, Wakeling A: Abnormal eating attitudes in London schoolgirls-a prospective epidemiological study: outcome a twelve month follow-up. Psychological Medicine 1990;20:383-394.

480. Kendler KS, MacLean C, Neale M, Kessler R, Heath A, Eaves L: The genetic epidemiology of bulimia nervosa. American Journal of Psychiatry 1991;149:1627-1637.

481. Klem ML, Wing RR, Simkin-Silverman L, Kuller LH: The psychological consequences of weight gain prevention in healthy, premenopausal women. International Journal of Eating Disorders 1997;21:167-174.

482. Presnell K, Stice E: An experimental test of the effect of weight-loss dieting on bulimic pathology: tipping the scales in a different direction. Journal of Abnormal Psychology 2003;112:166-170.

483. Wadden TA, Foster GD, Sarwer DB, Anderson DA, Gladis M, Sanderson RS, Letchak RV, Berkowitz RI, Phelan S: Dieting and the development of eating disorders in obese women: results of a randomized controlled trial. American Journal of Clinical Nutrition 2004;80:560-568.

484. National Task Force on the Prevention and Treatment of Obesity: Dieting and the development of eating disorders in overweight and obese adults. Archives of Internal Medicine 2000;160:2581-2589.

485. Wilson GT: Relation of Dieting and Voluntary Weight Loss to Psychological Functioning and Binge Eating. Annals of Internal Medicine 1993;119:727-730.

486. Chevrier J, Dewailly E, Ayotte P, Mauriege P, Despres JP, Tremblay A: Body weight loss increases plasma and adipose tissue concentrations of potentially toxic pollutants in obese individuals. International Journal of Obesity and Related Metabolic Disorders 2000;24:1272-1278.

487. Braune B, Muir D, DeMarch B, Gamberg M, Poole K, Currie R, Dodd M, Duschenko W, Eamer J, Elkin B, Evans M, Grundy S, Hebert C, Johnstone R, Kidd K, Koenig B, Lockhart L, Marshall H, Reimer K, Sanderson J,

Shutt L: Spatial and temporal trends of contaminants in Canadian Arctic freshwater and terrestrial ecosystems: a review. Science of the Total Environment 1999;230:145-207.

488. Pelletier C, Imbeault P, Tremblay A: Energy balance and pollution by organochlorines and polychlorinated biphenyls. Obesity Reviews 2003;4:17-24.

489. Rodin J, Radke-Sharp N, Rebuffe-Scrive M, Greenwood MR: Weight cycling and fat distribution. International Journal of Obesity 1990;14:303-310.

490. Williamson DF: "Weight cycling" and mortality: how do epidemiologists explain the role of intentional weight loss? Journal of the American College of Nutrition 1996;15:6-13.

491. Albu J, Smolowitz J, Lichtman S, Heymsfield SB, Wang J, Pierson JrRN, Pi-Sunyer FX: Composition of Weight Loss in Severely Obese Women:A New Look at Old Methods. Metabolism 1992;41:1068-1074.

492. Everhart JE: Contributions of Obesity and Weight Loss to Gallstone Disease. Annals of Internal Medicine 1993;119:1029-1035.

493. Weinsier RL, Wilson LJ, Lee J: Medically safe rate of weight loss for the treatment of obesity: a guideline based on risk of gallstone formation. American Journal of Medicine 1995;98:115-117.

494. Riedt CS, Cifuentes M, Stahl T, Chowdhbury HA, Schlussel Y, Shapses SA: Overweight postmenopausal women lose bone with moderate weight reduction and 1 g/day calcium intake. Journal of Bone and Mineral Research 2005;20:455-463.

495. Ensrud KE, Fullman RL, Barrett-Connor E, Cauley JA, Stefanick ML, Fink HA, Lewis CE, Orwoll E, Study of Osteoporotic Fractures Research Group: Voluntary Weight Reduction in Older Men Increases Hip Bone Loss: The Osteoporotic Fractures in Men Study. Journal of Clinical Endocrinology and Metabolism 2005;90:1998-2004.

496. Ensrud KE, Ewing SK, Stone KL, Cauley JA, Bowman PJ, Cummings SR, Study of Osteoporotic Fractures Research Group: Intentional and unintentional weight loss increase bone loss and hip fracture risk in older women. Journal of the Geriatric Society 2003;51:1740-1747.

497. Langlois JA, Visser M, Davidovic LS, Maggi S, Guohua L, Harris TB: Hip Fracture Risk in Older White Men Is Associated with Change in Body Weight From Age 50 Years to Old Age. Archives of Internal Medicine 1998;158:990-996.

498. Villareal DT, Shah K, Banks MR, Sinacore DR, Klein S: Effect of Weight Loss and Exercise Therapy on Bone Metabolism and Mass in Obese Older Adults: A One-Year Randomized Controlled Trial. Journal of Clinical Endocrinology and Metabolism 2008;93:2181-2187.

499. Freedman MR, King J, Kennedy E: Popular Diets: A Scientific Review. Obesity Research 2001;9:1S-40S.

500. Trichopoulou A, Bamia C, Trichopoulou D: Mediterranean Diet and Survival Among Patients With Coronary Heart Disease in Greece. Archives of Internal Medicine 2005;165:929-935.

501. Trichopoulou A, EPIC-Elderly Prospective Study Group: Modified Mediterranean diet and survival: EPIC-elderly prospective cohort study. BMJ 2005;330:991-995.

502. Knoops KT, de Groot LC, Kromhout D, Perrin AE, Moreiras-Varela O, Menotti A, van Staveren WA: Mediterranean diet, lifestyle factors, and 10-year mortality in elderly European men and women: the HALE project. JAMA 2004;292:1490-1492.

503. Gifford KD: Dietary Fats, Eating Guides, and Public Policy: History, Critique, and Recommendations. American Journal of Medicine 2002;113:89S-106S.

504. Hill JO, Drougas H, Peters JC: Obesity Treatment: Can Diet Composition Play a Role? Annals of Internal Medicine 1993;119:694-697.

505. Kennedy ET, Bowman SA, Spence JT, Freedman M, King J: Popular diets: Correlation to health, nutrition, and obesity. Journal of the American Dietetic Association 2001;101:411-420.

506. Institute of Medicine. Dietary Reference Intakes for Energy, Carbohydrate, Fiber, Fat, Fatty Acids, Cholesterol, Protein, and Amino Acids. 2002. Washington D.C., National Academy Press. t

507. Dansiger ML, Gleason JA, Griffith JL, Selker HP, Schaefer F: Comparison of the Atkins, Ornish, Weight Watchers, and Zone Diets for Weight Loss and Heart Disease Risk Reduction. JAMA 2005;293:43-53.

508. Foster GD, Wyatt HR, Hill JO, McGuckin BG, Brill C, Mohammed BS, Szapary PO, Rader DJ, Edman JS, Klein S: A Randomized Trial of a Low Carbohydrate Diet for Obesity. New England Journal of Medicine 2003;348:2082-2090.

509. Gardner CD, Kiazand A, Alhassan S, Kim S, Stafford RS, Balise RR, Kraemer HC, King AC: Comparison of the Atkins, Zone, Ornish, and LEARN Diets for Change in Weighgt and Related Risk Factor Among Overweight Premenopausal Women. JAMA 2007;297:969-977.

510. Stern L, Iqbal N, Seshadri P, Chicano KL, Daily DA, McGrory J, Williams M, Gracely EJ, Samaha FF: The Effects of Low-Carbohydrate versus Conventional Weight Loss Diets in Severely Obese Adults: One year Follow-up of a Randomized Trial. Annals of Internal Medicine 2004;140:778-785.

511. The Truth about LOW-CARB FOODS. Consumers Reports , 12-15. 2004. Yonkers, NY, Consumers Union. 6-1-2004.

512. Feinman, R. D. and Fine, E. J. "A calorie is a calorie" violates the second law of thermodynamics. 2004.

513. Bisschop PH, Pereira Arias AM, Ackermans MT, Endert E, Pijl H, Kuipers F, Meijer AJ, Sauerwein HP, Romijn JA: The Effects of Carbohydrate Variation in Isocaloric Diets on Glycogenolysis and Gluconeogenesis in Healthy Men. Journal of Clinical Endocrinology and Metabolism 2000;85:1963-1967.

514. Jéquier E: Pathways to obesity. International Journal of Obesity and Related Metabolic Disorders 2002;26:S12-S7.

515. Johnston CS, Day CS, Swan PD: Postprandial Thermogenesis is increased 100% on a High-Protein, Low-Fat Diet versus a High-Carbohydrate, Low-Fat Diet in Healthy, Young Women. Journal of the American College of Nutrition 2002;21:55-61.

516. Dauncey MJ, Bingham SA: Dependence of 24 h energy expenditure in man on the composition of the nutrient intake. British Journal of Nutrition 1983;50:1-13.

517. Karst H, Steiniger J, Noack R, Steglich HD: Diet-induced thermogenesis in man: thermic effects of single proteins, carbohydrates and fats depending on their energy amount. Annals of Nutrition and Metabolism 1984;28:245-252.

518. Nair KS, Halliday D, Garrow JS: Thermic response to isoenergetic protein, carbohydrate or fat meals in lean and obese subjects. Clinical Science London 1983;65:307-312.

519. Robinson SM, Jaccard C, Persaud C, Jackson AA, Jequier E, Schutz Y: Protein turnover and thermogenesis in response to high-protein and high-carbohydrate feeding in men. American Journal of Clinical Nutrition 1990;52:72-80.

520. Bravata DM, Sanders L, Huang J, Krumholz HM, Olkin I, Gardner CD, Bravata DM: Efficacy and safety of low-carbohydrate diets: a systematic review. JAMA 2003;289:1837-1850.

521. Reddy ST, Wang CY, Sakhaee K, Brinkley L, Pak CY: Effect of low-carbohydrate high-protein diets on acid-base balance, stone-forming propensity, and calcium metabolism. American Journal of Kidney Disease 2002;40:265-274.

522. Fleming RM: The effect of high-protein diets on coronary blood flow. Angiology 2000;51:817-826.

523. D'Anci KE, Watts KL, Kanarek RB, Taylor HA: Low-carbohydrate weight-loss diets. Appetite 2009;52:96-103.

524. Halyburton AK, Brinkworth GD, Wilson CJ, Noakes M, Buckley JD, Keogh JB, Clifton PM: Low- and high-carbohydrate weight-loss diets have similar effects on mood but not cognitive performance. American Journal of Clinical Nutrition 2007;86:580-587.

525. Amatruda JM, Biddle TL, Patton ML, Lockwood DH: Vigorous supplementation of a hypocaloric diet prevents cardiac arrhythmias and mineral depletion. American Journal of Medicine 1983;74:1016-1022.

526. Wadden TA, Stunkard AJ, Brownell KD: Very low calorie diets: their efficacy, safety and future. Annals of Internal Medicine 1983;99:675-684.

527. National Task Force on the Prevention and Treatment of Obesity NIoH: Very low-calorie diets. JAMA 1993;270:967-974.

528. de Lorgeril M, Salen P, Martin J-L, Monjaud I, Delaye J, Mamelle N: Mediterranean Diet, Traditional Risk Factors, and the Rate of Cardiovascular Complications After Myocardial Infarction: Final Report of the Lyon Diet Heart Study. Circulation 1999;99:779-785.

529. Broom DR, Batterham RL, King JA, Stensel DJ: Influence of resistance and aerobic exercise on hunger, circulating levels of acylated ghrelin, and peptide YY in healthy males. American Journal of Physiology 2009;296:R29-R35.

530. Goodpaster BH, Wolfe RR, Kelley DE: Effect of Obesity on Substrate Utilization during Exercise. Obesity Research 2002;10:575-584.

531. Samaras K, Kelly PJ, Chiano MN, Spector TD, Campbell LV: Genetic and Environmental Influences on Total-Body and Central Abdominal Fat: The Effect of Physical Activity in Female Twins. Annals of Internal Medicine 1999;130:873-882.

532. Ross R, Dagnone D, Jones PJH, Smith H, Paddags A, Hudson R, Janssen I: Reduction in Obesity and Related Comorbid Conditions after Diet-Induced Weight- Loss or Exercise-Induced Weight Loss in Men. Annals of Internal Medicine 2000;133:92-103.

533. Slentz CA, Duscha BD, Johnson JL, Ketchum K, Aiken LB, Samsa GP, Houmard JA, Bales CW, Kraus WE: Effects of the amount of exercise on body weight, body composition, and measures of central obesity: STRRIDE-A RANDOMIZED CONTROLLED STUDY. Archives of Internal Medicine 2004;164:31-39.

534. Schoeller DA, Shay K, Kushner RF: How much physical activity is needed to minimize weight gain in previously obese women? American Journal of Clinical Nutrition 1997;66:551-556.

535. Jakicic JM, Winters C, Lang W, Wing RR: Effects of Intermittent Exercise and Use of Home Exercise Equipment on Adherence, Weight Loss, and Fitness in Overweight Women. JAMA 1999;282:1554-1560.

536. Bahr R, Sejersted OM: Effect of Intensity of Exercise on Excess Postexercise O_2 Consumption. Metabolism 1991;40:836-841.

537. Davidson MH, Hauptman J, DiGirolamo M, Foreyt JP, Halsted CH, Heber D, Heimburger DC, Lucas CP, Robbins DC, Chung J, Heymsfield SB: Weight Control and Risk Factor Reduction in Obese Subjects Treated for 2 Years With Orlistat. JAMA 1999;281:235-242.

538. James WPT, Astrup A, Finer N, Hilsted J, Kopelman P, Rössner S, Saris WHM, Gaal LCF: Effect of sibutramine on weight maintenance after weight loss: a randomised trial. Lancet 2000;356:2119-2125.

539. Sjöström L, Rissanen A, Andersen T, Boldrin M, Golay A, Koppeschaar HPF, Krempf M: Randomised placebo-controlled trial of orlistat for weight loss and prevention of weight regain in obese patients. Lancet 1998;352:167-172.

540. McNeely W, Benfield P: Orlistat. Drugs 1998 1998;56:241-249.

541. Weigle DS: Pharmacological Therapy of Obesity: Past, Present, and Future. Journal of Clinical Endocrinology and Metabolism 2003;88:2462-2469.

542. Li Z, Maglione M, Tu W, Mojica W, Arterburn D, Shugarman LR, Hilton L, Suttorp M, Solomon V, Shekelle PG, Morton SC: Meta-Analysis: Pharmacologic Treatment of Obesity. Annals of Internal Medicine 2005;142:532-546.

543. Snow V, Barry P, Fitterman N, Qaseem A, Weiss K: Pharmacologic and Surgical Management of Obesity in Primary Care: A Clinical Practice Guideline from the American College of Physicians. Annals of Internal Medicine 2005;142:525-531.

544. NIH Technology Assessment Conference Panel: METHODS FOR VOLUNTARY WEIGHT LOSS AND CONTROL. Annals of Internal Medicine 1993;119:764-770.

545. Wadden TA, Butryn ML, Byrne KJ: Efficacy of Lifestyle Modification for Long-Term Weight Control. Obesity Research 2004;12:151S-162S.

546. Shaw, K., O'Rourke, P., Del Mar, C., and Kenardy, J. Psychological interventions for overweight or obesity. 2. 2005. John Wiley & Sons, Ltd.

547. Wadden TA, Sternberg JA, Letizia KA, Stunkard AJ, Foster GD: Treatment of obesity by very low calorie diet, behavior therapy, and their combination: a five-year perspective. International Journal of Obesity 1989;13:39-46.

548. Douketis JD, Feightner JW, Attia J, Feldman WF: Periodic health examination, 1999 update: 1. Detection, prevention and treatment of obesity. Canadian Medical Association Journal 1999;160:513-525.

549. McTigue KM, Harris R, Hemphill B, Lux L, Sutton S, Bunton AJ, Lohr KN: Screening and Interventions for Obesity in Adults: Summary of the Evidence for the U.S. Services Task Force. Annals of Internal Medicine 2003;139:933-949.

550. Foster GD, Wadden TA, Phelan S, Sarwer DB, Sanderson RS: Obese Patients' Perceptions of Treatment Outcomes and the factors that Influence Them. Archives of Internal Medicine 2001;161:2133-2139.

551. Staff of the Federal Trade Commission. Deception in Weight-Loss Advertising Workshop: Seizing Opportunities and Building Partnerships to Stop Weight-Loss Fraud. 2003. Rockville, MD, Office of the Surgeon General.

552. Serdula MK, Mokdad AH, Williamson DF, Galuska DA, Mendlein JW, Heath GW: Prevalence of Attempting Weight Loss and Strategies for Controlling Weight. JAMA 1999;282:1353-1358.

553. Flegal KM, Carroll MD, Ogden CL, Johnson CL: Prevalence and Trends in Obesity Among US Adults, 1999-2000. JAMA 2002;288:1723-1727.

554. Hedley AA, Ogden CL, Johnson CL, Carroll MD, Curtin LR, Flegal KM: Prevalence of Overweight and Obesity Among US Children, Adolescents, and Adults, 1999-2000. JAMA 2006;291:2847-2850.

555. Expert Panel, National Institutes of Health. The Practical Guide Identification, Evaluation, and Treatment of Overweight and Obesity in Adults. 1-80. 2000. National Heart, Lung and Blood Institute.

556. Wing RR, Phelan S: Long-term weight loss maintenance. American Journal of Clinical Nutrition 2005;82S:222S-225S.

557. Delparigi, A., Chen, K., Salbe, A.D., Hill, J.O., Wing, R.R., Reiman, E.M., and Tataranni, P.A. Successful dieters have increased neural activity in cortical areas involved in the control of behavior. International Journal of Obesity. 2006.

558. Nicklas TA, Baranowski T, Cullen KW, Berenson G: Eating Patterns, Dietary Quality and Obesity. Journal of the American College of Nutrition 2001;20:599-608.

559. Williams DE, Cadwell BL, Cheng YJ, Cowie CC, Gregg EW, Geiss LS, Engelgau MM, Narayan KM, Imperatore G: Prevalence of impaired fasting glucose and its relationship with cardiovascular disease risk factors in US adolescents 1999-2000. Pediatrics 2005;116:1122-1126.

560. Olshansky SJ, Passaro DJ, Hershow RC, Layden J, Carnes BA, Brody J, Hayflick L, Butler RN, Allison DB, Ludwig DS: A Potential Decline in Life Expectancy in the United States in the 21st Century. New England Journal of Medicine 2005;352:1138-1145.

561. Summerbell, C. D., Waters, E., Edmunds, L. D., Kelly, S., Brown, T., and Campbell, K. J. Interventions for preventing obesity in children. 2005. University of Teesside, UK. Cochrane Database Systematic Reviews.

562. Kalarchian MA, Levine MD, Arslanian SA, Ewing LJ, Houck PR, Cheng Y, Ringham RM, Sheets CA, Marcus MD: Family-Based Treatment of Severe Pediatric Obesity: Randomized, Controlled Trial. Pediatrics 2009;124:1060-1068.

563. Belkin, L. The School-Lunch Test. New York Times Magazine. 8-20-2006.

564. US Preventive Services Task Force: Screening and Interventions for Overweight in Children and Adolescents: Recommendation Statement. Pediatrics 2005;116:205-209.

565. Sturm R: Increases in Clinically Severe Obesity. Archives of Internal Medicine 2003;163:2146-2148.

566. Nguyen NT, Wilson SE: Complications of antiobesity surgery. Nature Clinical Practise Gastroenterology & Hepatology 2007;4:138-147.

567. Phurrough, S., Salive, M. E., Brechner, R. J., Tillman, K., Harrison, S., and O'Connor, D. Decision Memo for Bariatric Surgery for the Treatment of Morbid Obesity (CAG-00250R). 2006. Centers for Medicare & Medicaid Services.

568. Inge TH, Xanthakos SA, Zeller MH: Bariatric surgery for pediatric extreme obesity: now or later? International Journal of Obesity 2007;31:1-14.

569. Couzin J: Bypassing Medicine to Treat Obesity. Science 2008;320:438-440.

570. Herron DM: The Surgical Management of Severe Obesity. Mount Sinai Journal of Medicine 2004;71:63-71.

571. Presutti RJ, Gorman S, Swain JM: Primary Care Perspective on Bariatric Surgery. Mayo Clinic Proceedings 2004;79:1158-1166.

572. Strader AD, Vahl TP, Jandacek RJ, Woods SC, D'Alessio DA, Seeley RJ: Weight loss through ileal transposition is accompanied by increased ileal hormone secretion and synthesis in rats. American Journal of Physiology Endocrinology and Metabolism 2005;288:E447-E453.

573. Le Roux CW, Aylwin SJB, Batterham RL, Borg CM, Coyle F, Prasad V, Shurey S, Ghatei MA, Patel AG, Bloom SR: Gut Hormone Profiles Following Bariatric Surgery Favor an Anorectic State, Facilitate Weight Loss, and Improve Metabolic Parameters. Annals of Surgery 2006;243:108-114.

574. Morínigo R, Moizé V, Musri M, Lacy AM, Navarro S, Marín JL, Delgado S, Casamitjana R, Vidal J: Glucagon-Like Peptide-1, Peptide YY, Hunger, and Satiety after Gastric Bypass Surgery in Morbidly Obese Subjects. Journal of Clinical Endocrinology and Metabolism 2006;91:1735-1740.

575. DeMaria EJ, Murr M, Byrne TK, Blackstone R, Grant JP, Budak A, Wolfe L: Validation of the obesity surgery mortality risk score in a multicenter study proves it stratifies mortality risk in patients undergoing gastric bypass for morbid obesity. Annals of Surgery 2007;246:578-582.

576. Christou NV, Sampalis JS, Liberman M, Look D, Auger S, McLean APH, McLean LD: Surgery Decreases Long-term Mortality, Morbidity, and Health Care Use in Morbidly Obese Patients. Annals of Surgery 2004;240:416-424.

577. Flum DR, Dellinger EP: Impact of gastric bypass operation on survival: a population-based analysis. Journal of American College of Surgeons 2004;199:543-551.

578. MacDonald KGJr, Long SG, Swanson MS, Brown BM, Morris P, Dohm GL, Pories WJ: The Gastric Bypass Operation Reduces the Progression and Mortality of Non-Insulin-Dependent Diabetes Mellitus. Journal of Gastrointestinal Surgery 1997;1:213-220.

579. Sjöström L, Narbro K, Sjöström CD, Karason K, Larsson B, Wedel H, Lystig T, Sullivan M, Bouchard C, Carlson B, Bengtsson C, Dahlgren S, Gummesson A, Jacobson P, Karlsson J, Lindroos A-K, Lönroth H, Näslund I, Olbers T, Stenlöf K, Torgerson J, Ågren G, Carlsson LMS: Effects of Bariatric Surgery on Mortality in Swedish Obese Subjects. New England Journal of Medicine 2007;357:741-752.

580. Adams TD, Gress RE, Smith SC, Halverson RC, Simper SC, Rosamond WD, LaMonte MJ, Stroup AM, Hunt SC: Long-Term Mortality after Gastric Bypass Surgery. New England Journal of Medicine 2007;357:753-761.

581. Hollis S, Campbell F: What is meant by intention to treat analysis? Survey of published randomised controlled trials. BMJ 1999;319:670-674.

582. Skelton, J. A., Cook, S. R., Auinger, P., Klein, J. D., and Barlow, S. E. Prevalence and Trends of Severe Obesity Among US Children and Adolescents. Academic Pediatrics . 2009.

583. Hammoud A, Gibson M, Hunt SC, Adams TD, Carrell DT, Kolotkin RL, Meikie AW: Effect of Roux-en-Y gastric bypass surgery on sex steroids and quality of life in obese men. Journal of Clinical Endocrinology and Metabolism 2009;94:1329-1332.

584. Sjöström L, Gummesson A, Sjöström CD, Narbro K, Peltonen M, Wedel H, Bengtsson C, Bouchard C, Carlsson B, Dahlgren S, Jacobson P, Karason K, Karlsson J, Larsson B, Lindroos AK, Lönroth H, Näslund I, Olbers T, Stenlöf K, Torgerson J, Carlsson LM, Swedish Obese Subjects Study: Effects of bariatric surgery on cancer incidence in obese patients in Sweden (Swedish Obese Subjects Study): a prospective controlled intervention trial. Lancet Oncology 2009;10:653-662.

585. Trus TL, Pope GD, Finlayson SR: National trends in utilization and outcomes of bariatric surgery. Surgical Endoscopy 2005;19:616-620.

586. Pope GD, Birkmeyer JD, Finlayson SR: National trends in utilizationn and in-hospital outcomes of bariatric surgery. Journal of Gastrointestinal Surgery 2002;6:855-860.

587. Santry HP, Gillen DL, Lauderdale DS: Trends in Bariatric Surgical Procedures. JAMA 2005;294:1909-1917.

588. Sjöström L, Lindroos A-K, Peltonen L, Torgerson J, Bouchard C, Carlson B, Dahlgren S, Larsson B, Narbro K, Sjöström CD, Sullivan M, Wedel H: Lifestyle, Diabetes, and Cardiovascular Risk Factors 10 Years after Bariatric Surgery. New England Journal of Medicine 2004;351:2683-2693.

589. Benotti PN, Forse A: The Role of Gastric Surgery in the Multidisciplinary Management of Severe Obesity. American Journal of Surgery 1995;169:361-367.

590. McLean LD, Rhode BM, Nohr CW: Late Outcome of Isolated Gastric Bypass. Annals of Surgery 2000;231:524-528.

591. Buchwald H, Avidor Y, Braunwald E, Jensen MD, Pories W, Fahrbach K, Schoelles K: Bariatric Surgery A Systematic Review and Meta-Analysis. JAMA 2004;292:1724-1737.

592. Colquitt, J. L., Picot, J., Loveman, E., and Clegg, A. J. Surgery for obesity. Cochrane Database of Systematic Reviews (2). 2009.

593. Pories WJ, Swanson MS, MacDonald KG, Long SB, Morris PG, Brown BM, Barakat H, deRamon RA, Israel G, Dolezal JM: Who would have thought it? An operation proves to be the most effective therapy for adult-onset diabetes. Annals of Surgery 1995;222:339-352.

594. Schauer PR, Burguera BG, Ikramuddin S, Cottam D, Gourash W, Hamad G, Eid GM, Mattar S, Ramanathan R, Barinas-Mitchel E, Rao RH, Kuller L, Kelley D: Effect of Laparoscopic Roux-En Y Gastric Bypass on Type 2 Diabetes Mellitus. Annals of Surgery 2003;238:467-485.

595. Sugerman HJ, Wolfe LG, Sica DA, Clorer JN: Diabetes and Hypertension in Severe Obesity and Effects of Gastric Bypass-induced Weight Loss. Annals of Surgery 2003;237:751-758.

596. Buchwald H, Estok R, Fahrbach K, Banel D, Jensen MD, Pories WJ, Bantle JP, Sledge I: Weight and type 2 diabetes after bariatric surgery: systematic review and meta-analysis. American Journal of Medicine 2009;122:248-256.

597. Sjöström CD, Lissner L, Wedel H, Sjöström L: Reduction in incidence of diabetes, hypertension and lipid disturbances after intentional weight loss induced by bariatric surgery: the SOS Intervention Study. Obesity Research 1999;7:477-484.

598. Coates PS, Fernstrom JD, Fernstrom MH, Schauer PR, Greenspan SL: Gastric Bypass Surgery for Morbid Obesity Leads to an Increase in Bone Turnover and a Decrease in Bone Mass. Journal of Clinical Endocrinology and Metabolism 2004;89:1061-1065.

599. Clancy TE, Moore FDJr, Zinner MJ: Post-gastric bypass hyperinsulinism with nesidioblastosis: subtotal or total pancreatectomy may be needed to prevent recurrent hypoglycemia. Gastrointestinal Surgery 2006;10:1116-1119.

600. Goldfine AB, Mun EC, Devine E, Bernier R, Baz-Hecht M, Jones DB, Schneider BE, Holst JJ, Patti ME: Patients with Neuroglycopenia after Gastric Bypass Surgery Have Exaggerated Incretin and Insulin Secretory Responses to a Mixed Meal. Journal of Clinical Endocrinology and Metabolism 2007;92:4678-4685.

601. Patti ME, McMahon G, Mun EC, Bitton A, Holst JJ, Goldsmith J, Hanto DW, Callery M, Arky R, Bonner-Weir S, Goldfine AB: Severe hypoglycemia post-gastric bypass requiring partial pancreatectomy: evidence for inappropriate insulin secretion and pancreatic islet hyperplasia. Diabetologia 2005;48:2236-2240.

602. Compston JE, Vedi S, Ledger JE, Webb A, Gazet J-C, Pilkington TRE: Vitamin D Status and bone histomorphometry in gross obesity. American Journal of Clinical Nutrition 1981;34:2359-2363.

603. Ågren G, Narbro K, Jonsson E, Näslund I, Sjöström L, Peltonen M: Cost of In-Patient Care over 7 Years among Surgically and Conventionally Treated Obese Patients. Obesity Research 2002;10:1276-1283.

604. Narbro K, Agren G, Jonsson E, Naslund T, Sjöström L, Peltonen M, Swedish Obese Subjects Intervention Study: Pharmaceutical costs in obese individuals: comparison with a randomly selected population sample and long-term changes after conventional and surgical treatment: the SOS intervention study. Archives of Internal Medicine 2002;162:2061-2069.

605. Sampalis JS, Liberman M, Auger S, Christou NV: The impact of weight reduction surgery on health-care costs in morbidly obese patients. Obesity Surgery 2004;14:939-947.

606. Clegg A, Colquitt J, Sidhu M, Royle P, Walker A: Clinical and cost effectiveness of surgery for morbid obesity: a systematic review and economic evaluation. International Journal of Obesity and Related Metabolic Disorders 2003;27:1167-1177.

607. Craig BM, Tseng DS: Cost-effectiveness of Gastric Bypass for Severe Obesity. American Journal of Medicine 2002;113:491-498.

608. Fang J: The cost-effectiveness of bariatric surgery. American Journal of Gastroenterology 2003;98:2097-2098.

609. Martin LF, Tan TL, Horn JR, Bixler EO, Kauffman GL, Becker DA, Hunter SM: Comparison of the costs associated with medical and surgical treatment of obesity. Surgery 1995;118:599-606.

610. Salem L, Jensen CC, Flum DR: Are Bariatric Surgical Outcomes Worth Their Cost? A Systematic Review. Journal of American College of Surgeons 2005;200:270-278.

611. Khan LK, Sobush K, Keener D, Goodman K, Lowry A, Kakietek J, Zaro S: Recommended Community Strategies and Measurements to Prevent Obesity in the United States. MMWR Recommendations and Reports 2009;58(RR07):1-26.

612. Troiano RP, Flegal KM: Overweight Children and Adolescents: Description, Epidemiology, and Demographics. Pediatrics 1998;101:497-504.

613. Cokkinides V, Bandi P, Ward E, Jemal A, Thun M: Progress and Opportunities in Tobacco Control. CA: A Cancer Journal for Clinicians 2006;56:135-142.

614. Hill JO, Wyatt HR, Reed GW, Peters JC: Obesity and the Environment: Where Do We Go from Here. Science 2003;299:853-855.

615. Spivak CD: The specific gravity of the human body. Archives of Internal Medicine 1915;15:628-642.

616. Brozek J, Grande F, Anderson JT, Keys A: Densitometric Analysis of Body Composition: Revision of Some Quantitative Assumptions. Annals of the New York Academy of Sciences 1963;110:113-140.

617. Morales MF, Rathbun EN, Smith RE, Pace N: Studies on Body Composition II. Theoretical Considerations Regarding the Major Body Tissue Components with Suggestions for Application to Man. Journal of Biological Chemistry 1945;158:677-684.

618. Mitchell HH, Hamilton TS, Steggerda FR, Bean HW: The chemical composition of the adult human body and its bearing on the biochemistry of growth. Journal of Biological Chemistry 1945;158:625-637.

619. Allen TH, Welch BE, Trujillo TT, Roberts JE: Fat, water and tissue solids of the whole body less its bone mineral. Journal of Applied Physiology 1959;14:1009-1012.

620. Lifson N, Gordon GB, McClintock R: Measurement of Total Carbon Dioxide Production by Means of D_2O^{18}. Journal of Applied Physiology 1955;7:704-710.

621. Lifson N, McClintock R: Theory of Use of the Turnover Rates of Body Water for Measuring Energy and Material Balance. Journal of Theoretical Biology 1966;12:46-74.

622. Mazess RB, Cameron JR, Sorenson JA: Determining Body Composition by Radiation Absorption Spectrometry. Nature 1970;228:771-772.

623. Beshyah SA, Freemantle C, Thomas E, Murphy M, Johnston DG: Comparison of Measurements of Body Composition by Total Body Potassium, Bioimpedance Analysis, and Dual-Energy X-Ray Absorptiometry in Hypopituitary Adults Before and During Growth Hormone Treatment. American Journal of Clinical Nutrition 1995;61:1186-1194.

624. Gotfredsen A, Jensen J, Borg J, Christiansen C: Measurement of Lean Body Mass and Total Body Fat Using Dual Photon Absorptiometry. Metabolism 1986;35:88-93.

625. Heymsfield SB, Wang J, Heshka S, Kehayias J, Pierson JrRN: Dual-photon absorptiometry: comparison of bone mineral and soft tissue mass measurements in vivo with established methods. American Journal of Clinical Nutrition 1989;49:1283-1289.

626. Venkataraman PS, Ahluwalia BW: Total Bone Mineral Content and Body Composition by X-ray Densitometry in Newborns. Pediatrics 1992;90:767-770.

627. Kohrt W: Body composition by DXA: tried and true? Medicine and Science in Sports and Exercise 1995;27:1349-1353.

628. Johnson J, Dawson-Hughes B: Precision and Stability of Dual-Energy X-ray Absorptiometry Measurements. Calcified Tissue International 1991;49:174-178.

629. Sievänen HT, Oja P, Vuori I: Scanner-induced variability and quality assurance in longitudinal dual-energy x-ray absorptiometry measurements. Medical Physics 1994;21:1795-1805.

630. Fogelholm GM, Sievänen HT, van Marken Lichtenbelt WD, Westerterp KR: Assessment of Fat-Mass Loss During Weight Reduction in Obese Women. Metabolism 1997;46:968-975.

631. Going SB, Massett MP, Hall MC, Bare LA, Root PA, Williams DP, Lohman TG: Detection of small changes in body composition by dual-energy x-ray absorptiometry. American Journal of Clinical Nutrition 1993;57:845-850.

632. Formica C, Atkinson MG, Nyulasi I, McKay J, Heale W, Seeman E: Body Composition Following Hemodialysis: Studies Using Dual-Energy X-Ray Absorptiometry and Bioelectrical Impedance Analysis. Osteoporosis International 1993;3:192-197.

633. Horber FF, Thomi F, Casez JP, Fonteille J, Jaeger Ph: Impact of hydration status on body composition as measured by dual energy X-ray absorptiometry in normal volunteers and patients on hemodialysis. British Journal of Radiology 1992;65:895-900.

634. Brunton JA, Weiler HA, Atkinson SA: Improvement in the Accuracy of Dual Energy X-ray Absorptiometry for Whole Body and Regional Analysis of Body Composition: Validation Using Piglets and Methodologic Considerations in Infants. Pediatric Research 1997;41:590-596.

635. Ellis KJ, Shypailo RJ, Pratt JA, Pond WG: Accuracy of dual-energy x-ray absorptiometry for body composition measurements in children. American Journal of Clinical Nutrition 1994;60:660-665.

636. Elowsson P, Forslund AH, Mallmin H, Feuk U, Hansson I, Carlsten J: An Evaluation of Dual-Energy X-Ray Absorptiometry and Underwater Weighing to Estimate Body Composition by Means of Carcass Analysis in Piglets. Journal of Nutrition 1998;128:1543-1549.

637. Friedberg W, Faulkner DN, Snyder L, Darden EB, O'Brien K: Galactic Cosmic Radiation Exposure and Associated Health Risks for Air Carrier Crewmembers. Aviation, Space, and Environmental Medicine 1989;60:1108.

638. Tothill P, Avenell A, Love J, Reid DM: Comparisons between Hologic, Lunar, and Norland dual-energy X-ray absorptiometers and other techniques used for whole-body soft tissue measurements. European Journal of Clinical Nutrition 1994;48:781.

639. Economos CD, Nelson ME, Fiatarone MA, Dallal GE, Heymsfield SB, Wang J, Yasumura S, Vaswani AN, Russell-Aulet M, Pierson JrRN: A multi-center comparison of dual energy X-ray absorptiometers: In vivo and in vitro soft tissue measurement. European Journal of Clinical Nutrition 1997;51:312-317.

640. Kistcorp CN, Svendsen OL: Body Composition analysis by dual energy X-ray absorptiometry in female diabetics differ between manufacturers. European Journal of Clinical Nutrition 1997;51:449-454.

641. Pierson JrRN, Wang J, Thornton JC, Kotler DP, Heymsfield SB, Weber DA, Ma R: Bone Mineral and Body Fat Measurements by Two Absorptiometry Systems : Comparisons with Neutron Activation Analysis. Calcified Tissue International 1995;56:93-98.

642. Hirsch J, Gallian E: Methods for the determination of adipose cell size in man and animals. Journal of Lipid Research 1971;12:521-530.

643. Fidanza F, Keys A, Anderson JT: Density of Body Fat in Man and Other Mammals. Journal of Applied Physiology 1953;6:252-256.

644. Mendez J: Density and Composition of Mammalian Muscle. Metabolism 1960;9:184-188.

645. Mendez J, Keys A, Anderson JT, Grande F: Density of Fat and Bone Mineral of the Mammalian Body. Metabolism 1960;9:472-477.

646. Siri, W. Body composition from fluid spaces and density: an analysis of methods. University of California Radiation Laboratory Report 3349. 1956.

647. Chumlea WC, Guo S, Baumgartner RN, Siervogel RM: Determination of Body Fluid Compartments with Multiple Frequency Bioelectric Impedance; in Ellis KJ, Eastman JD (eds): Human Body Composition. New York, Plenum Press, 1993 pp 23-26.

648. Hoffer EC, Meador CK, Simpson DC: Correlation of Whole-Body Impedance with Total Body Water Volume. Journal of Applied Physiology 1969;27:531-534.

649. Janssen YJH, Deurenberg P, Roelfsema F: Using Dilution Techniques and Multifrequency Bioelectrical Impedance to Assess Both Total Body Water and Extracellular Water at Baseline and during Recombinant Human Growth Hormone (GH) Treatment in GH-Deficient Adults. Journal of Clinical Endocrinology and Metabolism 1997;82:3349-3355.

650. Kushner RF, Schoeller DA: Estimation of Total Body Water by Bioelectrical Impedance Analysis. American Journal of Clinical Nutrition 1986;44:417-424.

651. Kushner RF, Kunigk A, Alspaugh M, Andronis PT, Leitch CA, Schoeller DA: Validation of Bioelectrical-Impedance Analysis as a Measurement of Change in Body Composition in Obesity. American Journal of Clinical Nutrition 1990;52:219-223.

652. Segal KR, Burastero S, Chun A, Coronel P, Pierson JrRN, Wang J: Estimation of Extracellular and Total Body Water by Multiple-Frequency Bioelectrical-Impedance Measurement. American Journal of Clinical Nutrition 1991;54:26-29.

653. Piccoli A, Pillon L, Favaro E: Asymmetry of the Total Body Water Prediction Bias Using the Impedance Index. Nutrition 1997;13:438-441.

654. Pace N, Rathbun EN: Studies on Body Composition. III. The Body Water and Chemically Combined Nitrogen Content in Relation to Fat Content. Journal of Biological Chemistry 1945;158:685-691.

655. Lukaski HC, Johnson PE, Bolonchuk WW, Lykken GI: Assessment of Fat-Free Mass using Bioelectrical Impedance Measurements of the Human Body. American Journal of Clinical Nutrition 1985;41:810-817.

656. Segal KR, Gutin B, Presta E, Wang J, Van Itallie TB: Estimation of Human Body Composition by Electrical Impedance Methods: a Comparative Study. Journal of Applied Physiology 1985;58:1565-1571.

657. Diaz EO, Villar J, Immink M, Gonzales T: Bioimpedance or Anthropometry. European Journal of Clinical Nutrition 1989;43:129-137.

658. Fuller NJ, Elia M: Potential Use of Bioelectrical Impedance of the 'Whole Body' and of Body Segments for the Assessment of Body Composition: Comparison with Densitometry and Anthropometry. European Journal of Clinical Nutrition 1989;43:779-791.

659. Deurenberg P, van der Kooy K, Leenen R, Weststrate JA, Seidell JC: Sex and Age Specific Prediction Formulas for Estimating Body Composition from Bioelectic Impedance: a Cross-Validation Study. International Journal of Obesity 1991;15:17-25.

660. Houtkooper LB, Lohman TG, Going SB, Hall MC: Validity of Bioelectric Impedance for Body Composition Assessment in Children. Journal of Applied Physiology 1989;66:814-821.

661. Deurenberg P, Weststrate JA, van der Kooy K: Body Composition Changes Assessed by Bioelectrical Impedance Measurements. American Journal of Clinical Nutrition 1989;49:401-403.

662. Deurenberg P, Weststrate JA, Hautvast JGAJ: Changes in Fat-Free Mass during Weight Loss Measured by Bioelectrical Impedance and by Densitometry. American Journal of Clinical Nutrition 1989;49:33-36.

663. Ross R, Léger L, Martin P, Roy R: Sensitivity of Bioelectrical Impedance to Detect Changes in Human Body Composition. Journal of Applied Physiology 1989;67:1643-1648.

664. van der Kooy K, Leenen R, Deurenberg P, Seidell JC, Westerterp KR, Hautvast JGAJ: Changes in Fat-Free Mass in Obese Subjects after Weight Loss: a Comparison of Body Composition Measures. International Journal of Obesity 1992;16:675-683.

665. National Institutes of Health. Bioelectrical Impedance Analysis in Body Composition Measurement. NIH Technol Assess Statement Online. National Institutes of Health Technology Assessment Conference 15. 1994. National Institutes of Health.

666. Comtrad, Inc. Does your Scale Measure your Weight and Body Fat Accurately? New York Times Magazine, 35. 1998. 1-18-1998.

667. Omron, Inc. Measuring Body Fat with Dignity. Modern Medicine 66, 13. 1998. 98.

668. Livesey G, Elia M: Estimation of energy expenditure, net carbohydrate utilization, and net fat oxidation and synthesis by indirect calorimetry: evaluation of errors with special reference to the detailed composition of fuels. American Journal of Clinical Nutrition 1988;47:608-628.

669. Culebras JM, Moore FD: Total Body Water and the Exchangeable Hydrogen I. Theoretical Calculation of nonaqueous Exchangeable Hydrogen in Man. American Journal of Physiology 1977;232:R54-R59.

670. Kachigan SK: Multivariate Statistical Analysis, ed 2. New York, Radius Press, 1991.

671. Hoffman JG, Hempelmann LH: Estimation of whole-body radiation doses in accidental fission bursts. American Journal of Roentgenology and Radium Therapy 1957;77:144-160.

672. Gamertsfelder CC, Larson HV, Nielsen JF, Roesch WC, Watson EC: Dosimetry investigation of the recuplex criticality accident. Health Physics 1963;9:757-768.

673. Anderson J, Osborn SB, Tomlinson RWS, Newton D, Rundo J, Salmon L, Smith JW: Neutron activation analysis in man in vivo. Lancet 1964;2:1201-1205.

674. Knight GS, Beddoe AH, Streat SJ, Hill GL: Body composition of two human cadavers by neutron activation and chemical analysis. American Journal of Physiology 1986;250:E179-E185.

675. Chettle DR, Fremlin JH: Techniques of in vivo neutron activation analysis. Physics in Medicine and Biology 1984;29:1011-1043.

676. Ma R, Dilmanian FA, Rarback H, Stamatelatos IE, Meron M, Yasumura S, Weber DA, Lidofsky LJ, Pierson Jr RN: Recent upgrade of the in vivo neutron activation facility at Brookhaven National Laboratory; in Eastman JD (ed): Human Body Composition. New York, Plenum Press, 1993 pp 345-350.

677. Ma K, Pierson JrRN, Wang J, Thornton JC, Ma R: Reliability of in vivo neutron activation analysis for measuring body composition: Comparisons with tracer dilution and dual-energy x-ray absorptiometry. Journal of Laboratory and Clinical Medicine 1996;127:420-427.

678. Segal KR, Van Loan M, Fitzgerald PI, Hodgdon JA, Van Itallie TB: Lean Body Mass Estimation by Bioelectical Impedance Analysis: a Four-site Study. American Journal of Clinical Nutrition 1988;47:7-14.

679. Mazariegos M, Wang Z, Gallagher D, Baumgartner RN, Allison DB, Wang J, Heysmfield S: Differences Between Young and Old Females in the Five Levels of Body Composition and Their Relevance to the Two-Compartment Chemical Model. Journal of Gerontology 1994;49:M201-M208.

680. Womersley J, Durnin JVGA, Boddy K, Mahaffy M: Influence of Muscular Development, Obesity, and Age on the Fat-Free Mass of Adults. Journal of Applied Physiology 1976;41:223-229.

681. Corsa L, Jr., Olney JM, Jr., Steenburg RW, Ball MR, Moore FD: The measurement of exchangeable potassium in man by isotope dilution. Journal of Clinical Investigation 1950;29:1280-1295.

682. St Jeor ST, Howard BV, Prewitt TE, Bovee V, Bazzarre T, Eckel RH: Dietary Protein and Weight Reduction. Circulation 2001;104:1869-1874.

683. Tack J, Caenepeel P, De Wulf D, Bisschops R: Pathophysiology, diagnosis and management of postoperative dumping syndrome. Nature Reviews Gastroenterology & Hepatology 2009;6:583-590.

684. Doelle GC: The clinical picture of metabolic syndrome. Postgraduate Medicine 2004;116:30-36.

www.ingramcontent.com/pod-product-compliance
Lightning Source LLC
Chambersburg PA
CBHW081656270326
41933CB00017B/3190